Geraghty's Caring for Children
Third edition

Geraghty's Caring for Children

Third Edition

Maureen O'Hagan BEd, MSc, MIHE, RGN, NNEB
Director of Quality Assurance
Council for Awards in Children's Care and Education
St Albans, Hertfordshire

Baillière Tindall
London Philadelphia Toronto Sydney Tokyo

Baillière Tindall   24–28 Oval Road,
WB Saunders Company Ltd London NW1 7DX

The Curtis Center, Independence Square West,
Philadelphia, PA 19106–3399, USA

Harcourt Brace & Company
55 Horner Avenue, Toronto,
Ontario M8Z 4X6, Canada

Harcourt Brace & Company, Australia
30–52 Smidmore Street, Marrickville,
NSW 2204, Australia

Harcourt Brace & Company, Japan
Ichibancho Central Building, 22–1 Ichibancho
Chiyoda-ku, Tokyo 102, Japan

First published 1981
Second Edition 1988

A catalogue record for this book is available from the British Library

ISBN 0-7020-1918-6

Phototypeset by Phoenix Photosetting, Chatham, Kent
Printed in Great Britain by Bath Press Colourbooks, Glasgow

Contents

Foreword vii
Acknowledgements viii
Preface ix

Chapter 1 Working with Children 1
Chapter 2 Child Health 23
Chapter 3 Child Safety 54
Chapter 4 Diet and Nutrition 70
Chapter 5 Working with Babies 84
Chapter 6 Child Development 119
Chapter 7 Children's Play and Education 165

Helping Agencies and their Addresses 201

Index 211

Foreword

Geraghty's Caring for Children has always been a good book; now, from the hands of Maureen O'Hagan, it has become an exceptionally timely one.

Although concern for the wellbeing and education of the very young has been spreading and intensifying since the landmark legislation of the Children Act, 1989, it has failed to make the UK more child-friendly. Most public concern has been targeted on family breakdown rather than family support, and expressed in negative judgements of modern parenting rather than positive plans for the care of modern children.

If the UK is to become a better place for children it has to recognize that many babies and young children get much of their experience of care and learning in daycare settings. We have to foster positive partnerships between parents and other caring adults and take positive measures to raise the quality of all child care. *Caring for Children* does both. Maureen O'Hagan recognizes that it is always individuals rather than institutions who meet infants' needs, so the knowledge and competence of adults who interact with children in nursery groups or classrooms is as crucial as that of adults – including parents and parent figures – who care for children in private homes. Knowledge and competence are here for the taking, but although they are carefully dovetailed to NVQs and CACHE awards, *Caring for Children* goes beyond any narrow interpretation of child care training to foster the personal and professional education and development of early years workers at every stage. Whether you are changing a baby's nappy on the first day of your first job, or planning to be among the early candidates for an NVQ level 4, this book will help you to think about why you do what you do, and to do it with sensitivity and respect for children and in a spirit of collaboration with parents.

Penelope Leach

ACKNOWLEDGEMENTS

To Mike, Rodan, Cass and other family and friends for their tolerance of my neglect of them whilst I have been writing. Also Sarah James, my editor and friend who has supported me throughout this project.

PUBLISHER'S ACKNOWLEDGEMENTS

All photographs, except those on pages 109, 114, 154 and 187, were provided by Joss Reiver Bany © 1997 and feature the children, staff and parents of Lea View Community Nursery, Springfield, London E5: our grateful thanks to all involved. The photographs on pages 109 and 114, of Nathaniel and Bethany James, were provided by Sarah James.

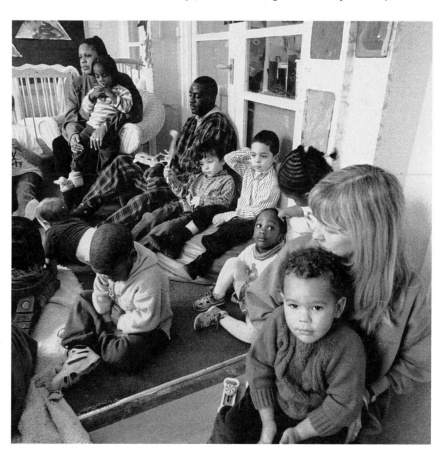

Preface

The First Edition of *Caring for Children* was written by Patricia Geraghty in 1981 and has proved to be a very popular book with child care workers and others who may wish to learn more about children. It was revised in 1988 and in 1990.

Having been asked by the publishers to provide a thorough revision of the book I set about looking at how things had changed since the last edition was written. A number of major changes have taken place in child care and education, the most significant being the Children Act 1989. This Act has been described as the most important piece of legislation this century. It united a number of previous Acts and made it very clear that the 'Welfare of the child is paramount'. Secondly, there has been a radical change in the way that child care and education workers are trained with the introduction of National Vocational Qualifications (NVQs). For the first time we have national standards for child care and education workers which demonstrate and legitimize the complexity and extensive knowledge required to carry out this work. National Vocational Qualifications in this field are at present only available at levels 2 and 3. However, it is expected that a level 4 will appear in the not too distant future.

The information in the First and Second Editions represented a great deal of underpinning knowledge and understanding which related to level 2 NVQs and it is for this reason that I have re-written the book to fit in with this level. At the same time we cannot ignore existing qualifications, the predominant of these being the awards offered by the Council for Awards in Children's Care and Education (CACHE) which incorporates the National Nursery Education Board (NNEB). In ordering the re-write I have tried to align the chapters with the NVQ system and the CACHE awards.

There is probably no single textbook which will provide all the information that a candidate or child care worker needs in order to gain the underpinning knowledge and understanding to enable them to do their job efficiently. However, '*Geraghty*' was traditionally a book which was able to offer both the health and education aspects and I have continued with that tradition.

Whilst writing the book, rapid changes have also taken place with regard to the early years curricula. The present government is piloting a voucher system for all 4-year-olds and as part of this they have introduced 'Desirable Learning Outcomes' for children entering compulsory education. At this moment we have no idea whether the voucher system will have a life beyond the piloting stage; however, I do not think that the 'Desirable Learning Outcomes' devised by the Schools Curriculum and Assessment Authority (SCAA) will disappear as they are very important in demonstrating the importance of the activities that take place in the pre-school setting. Another aspect that has to be considered is the consumer market: parents/carers are better informed and are able to 'shop around' for the best possible facility for their child. This has put child care and education into the competitive market, which means that issues of quality provision have come to the fore. Parents/carers are looking for quality provision, which amongst other things is able to demonstrate that the staff have had, or are receiving, a high level of training. If the voucher system is implemented nationally then all parents of 4-year-olds will become consumers, looking for the best quality of care for their child.

The layout of the book has been devised on a 'user friendly' basis and offers clear indications at the beginning of each chapter as to the NVQ units or CACHE award modules which the information in the chapter relates to. Each chapter has scenarios and assignments which the candidate can complete as part of their portfolio work and an extensive reference and further reading list on the areas covered by the chapter.

Finally, I hope that you will enjoy the book and find it useful to your studies.

Chapter 1

Working With Children

This chapter links with the following units for the National Vocational Qualifications (NVQs) in Child Care and Education: The underlying principles which underpin good practice.

INTRODUCTION

All those wishing to work with children need to have the knowledge and understanding of the child's wider role as a member of a family. There is a need to understand the different patterns of families and how these work as social units. Historically, the role of the child within society has moved from the child being treated as a mini-adult with no feelings (15th–16th century) through to the present day where the needs of the child are paramount (late 20th century). Such changes reflect the way that society has changed and evolved.

Child care workers also need to work in partnership with parents or the child's primary care-giver in order to ensure that all the child's needs are met. This requires the child care worker to have an understanding of family life and the factors which mitigate against families such as poverty, unemployment, racism, prejudice etc. Child care workers need to help build the parents' confidence by ensuring that they know that the child is safe in their care. In order to promote good practice, child care workers need to be understanding of children and adults, non-judgemental and committed to offering high quality child care and education. There is no official 'Code of Practice' for child care workers but the National Occupational Standards for Working with the Under Sevens and their Families has the following set of underlying principles which underpin good practice when working with children and their families:

◆ Demonstrating a caring and considerate attitude to children and parents
◆ Recognizing the crucial role that parents play and working in partnership with parents wherever possible
◆ Meeting all aspects of children's developmental needs
◆ Treating and valuing children as individuals

◆ Enabling children to be directors of their own learning
◆ Promoting equality of opportunity
◆ Celebrating cultural diversity
◆ Using language that is accessible and appropriate
◆ Sharing information and liaising with parents and other professionals
◆ Ensuring the health and safety of children and others

All good practice in child care work is based upon these underlying principles.

Present day society in the UK is culturally pluralistic, this means that it is made up of people from many cultures and religions. For the child care worker the most important point when dealing with children is that there is a duty to ensure that all the needs of each child are met, regardless of their, age, gender, ethnicity, religion or ability/disability. This is the basis of all good child care practice. This chapter will examine different family structures, factors which mitigate against families and the anti-discriminatory practices which all child care and education workers need to incorporate into their own practice.

DIFFERENT TYPES OF FAMILY

The family unit is a microcosm of the wider society, in other words it is a mini-reflection of the wider society. When a child lives with a family it will be introduced by the family to the values and norms of the wider society. Children will believe that the way things are done in their family is the way all families do things. It is only when they get older and visit other children's homes that they may realize that there are differences between families. It is important that child care workers do not undermine a child's family for however awful it may appear to the adult it is a very crucial part of a child's life.

The Extended Family

The *Collins Dictionary of Sociology* defines the extended family as:

> A group of people, related by kinship, where more than two generations of relatives live together (or in close proximity), usually forming a single household

The most famous study of extended families in the UK was carried out by Young and Wilmott (1962) when they looked at family life in Bethnal Green in East London during the 1950s. If you read this book it will give you some idea of how extended families in Britain operated. However, due to changes in housing and people moving around the country in order to find work there are very few extended families of the Young and Wilmott type left in the UK.

In order to study the extended family in present times it is necessary to look beyond the UK to countries such as Asia, Africa and South America.

Children born into the extended family will have the advantage of being able to bond with a number of adults who are all likely to take a part in the child rearing process. Studies have shown that within the extended family it is the women who have the strongest networks helping each other with tasks such as child care, cooking, shopping, doing the laundry and other domestic tasks. Much of the decision making is undertaken by the whole family and is based upon what is best for the family as a whole, not necessarily on what is best for the individual.

Extended families protect their members, and if there is a crisis it is most likely that family members will be consulted before help is sought from outside agencies. It is a close knit situation which offers advantages and disadvantages to its members.

Many people have found strength in being a member of an extended family as they are able to have support and help whenever they need it. Children are cared for within the broader family network, and it offers care and support to all its members. It is particularly useful for new parents and the elderly.

However, some people have found this type of family situation too suffocating as it inhibits individuality and privacy. Extended families place great pressure upon their members to conform to the family norms and values, and this can lead to conflict situations.

The Nuclear Family

The nuclear family is a small unit consisting of two adults and their children. It is the commonest form of family unit now found in the UK and Europe. With high divorce rates it is also very common to find that one of the adults may be a step-parent. Burgoyne and Clark (1982) estimated that in the UK, 7% of all children under the age of 17 years live with a step-parent. It is also quite common to find a couple living together with their children without being married.

Within an industrial society the nuclear family is the most economical type of living unit. It requires small living accommodation and offers independence from parents and other family members. It enables the family to move around the country easily in order to follow their work.

Within the nuclear family the adults are able to decide which of the wider family relations they will keep contact with and how frequently they will meet as a wider family. Nuclear families restrict the number of adults who are available for the child to relate to and in many instances prevent aunts, uncles and grandparents from taking a role in the child rearing process. Whilst the nuclear family is able to offer advantages in our present day society, it has also been blamed by politicians and others for a lot of the problems which have arisen in families, such as the high incidence of divorce, family violence and child abuse. Many nuclear families do not have the support of relatives close by who can help out in times of need; this puts an added stress upon the adults in the family who may be struggling to cope.

Lone Parent Families

According to Moss (1988), one in 10 households with a child under 10 years of age were lone parent families. A family may only have one parent due to death of one of the parents, separation, divorce or a woman producing a child outside of a relationship. Moss (1988), in his study of families in the 12 member states of the European Economic Union, found that the UK had the highest figures for divorce. This in turn led to a large number of lone parent families in the UK. Families where one of the parents is serving a prison sentence experience the same problems as other lone parent families.

Lone parents often find themselves in isolated positions with little or no support from members of their immediate family, who may live too far away to be of any assistance on a daily basis. Many lone parent families have to rely on income support as they are unable to work if they have small children. If they do manage to find part-time employment it is usually poorly paid and does not always cover the high costs that they may have to pay for child care. It must be remembered that not all lone parent families are 'problem families' and therefore do not qualify for a place for their child in a day nursery or other local authority supported provision. One of the greatest problems for lone parent families is trying to bring up a family on a low income; many families struggle to keep poverty at bay.

Reconstituted Families

This is the term that is used to describe the situation when two divorced people marry and form a family unit. With the very high divorce rate in the UK, this type of family is a very common social unit. Two previously married people coming together may result in them both becoming step-parents to children from the previous marriages. It may bring two groups of children into one family and there may also be children from the second marriage.

In many cases this type of family can work very well, but in some cases there may be resentment, rivalry and rancour that lead to stress and tension within the family. Being a step-parent is not an easy task and can be particularly difficult if the person has children of their own.

They will need to make a conscious effort not to put their own children's needs before the needs of the step-children. Step-parents have not in the past had good images in children's stories where they are often depicted as nasty, ugly and cruel (you only have to think of Cinderella). Many traditional stories have based their plot upon the theme of the wicked step-parent (usually step-mother). From such stories young children may have a very distorted view of what step-parents are like and this may cause them fear and distress. Children may also be resentful of the person who has displaced their real mother or father who they are now only able to see at weekends and holidays. Step-parents have to make very conscious efforts in order to build up relationships with their step-children. Step-parenting requires a great deal of sensitivity and understanding, and an acknowledgement that on many occasions they will find themselves in a 'no win' situation.

FACTORS WHICH MITIGATE AGAINST FAMILIES

Social Class and Home Life

The influence of the home upon the child has long lasting effects. It is the major influence upon the child during its first years of life. The effects of social class upon child rearing practices were clearly illustrated in a number of research projects carried out by John and Elizabeth Newsom in the late 1960s (Newsom and Newsom, 1976). More recently, Barbara Tizard *et al* (1988) in *Young Children at School in the Inner City* examined, amongst other things, the class factor and its relationship to those children who were underachievers.

The value system of the home will determine the way the family will rear its children. For example, the aristocracy use nannies as a preparation for the child going away to public school, whereas the middle classes may use nannies in order to enable the mother to continue her career. Research has shown that the middle classes make maximum use of pre-school facilities, whilst the working classes may feel that preparation for education is a waste of time as it has done nothing to help them in their search for a better lifestyle. However, it is significant that research has also shown that densely populated inner city working class areas are often poorly serviced with pre-school facilities, so working class parents who do value pre-school education may not have the facilities available to their children.

The home determines the language that the child will speak and the value system that the child will be introduced to. Basil Bernstein undertook considerable research in this area and put forward the theory that there are two language codes, the elaborated code, which is not context bound and is easily understood by all, and the restricted code, which is context bound and therefore difficult to understand outside the context to which it refers. Bernstein associated these codes with class stratification but other researchers have found that all people operate between the two codes. In some cases a child's home language may not be English and many under-fives are very successfully bilingual, moving easily between the language of the home and the language of the wider society.

The family of a child will determine which toys the child is given to play with, where they are taken on outings, whom they play with or are friends with etc. The family will also decide whether activities are undertaken as a family group, on an individual basis or whether older siblings are responsible for organizing the activities for the younger members of the family. Parental expectations also have a significant effect upon children's development. Such expectations range from the way a child behaves in different situations to what clothes they will be expected to wear, what activities they will participate in and how they progress through the education system.

The economic circumstances of the family will often have a bearing on the type of activities that a child may participate in. If the family has a car and money to spare, then outings will often happen on a regular basis and be away from the immediate home environment. Using public transport with small children can be a very daunting task, particularly for lone parents, and in these families activities are likely to take place closer to home.

Poverty

Poverty can affect families from all different social classes. We live in a society which is consumer orientated and one is only able to consume if the money is available. Oppenheim (1993) points out that '... poverty is about social exclusion imposed by an inadequate income. It is not only about having to go short of food or clothing, it is also about not being able to join a local sports club, or send your children on a school trip, or go out with friends or have a Christmas dinner.' Kumar (1993) states that in 1991 nearly one in every three children in the country were living in poverty. Not all poverty is due to unemployment: in a large number of cases, parents have employment but they earn far below the national average; others are sick or have disabilities which prevent them from working. However, unemployment has been a major cause of poverty amongst the middle classes who had what they thought were secure jobs for life within professions such as banking, accountancy, marketing etc. Many of these people have had their homes re-possessed by mortgage companies and have had to undergo a very drastic change in lifestyle. As the unemployment figures rise, so do the numbers of children that find themselves in poor households. Nina Oldfield in 1991 found that the weekly cost of a child was on average:

> £56.50 for a child aged 4 or 10 and £57.82 for a child aged 10 or 16 assuming that his/her parents are local authority tenants.
> £58.54 for a child aged 4 or 10 and £59.72 for a child aged 10 or 16 living in owner-occupied accommodation.
> (Quoted in Oppenheim, 1993, p. 62)

Whilst there are government benefits for those people who are low paid such as Family Income Supplement (FIS) or Family Credit (FC), these amounts are only intended to bring the low income up to the poverty line.

The effects that poverty has upon families are many, not least being the loss of self-esteem and worth as useful members of society and a poor quality of life. Bradshaw (1990) offers the following list of the impact and long term consequences of poverty on children:

◆ Physical which include
 - Infant mortality
 - Childhood deaths
 - Child morbidity
 - Child development
   Height
   Weight
   Nutrition
 - Racial disadvantage
 - Homelessness and housing conditions
 - Clothing
 - Child protection
 - Child abuse
◆ Behavioural which include
 - Education
 - Truancy
 - Teenage conceptions
 - Pocket money
 - Child labour
 - TV viewing
 - Smoking
 - Drinking
 - Drugs
 - Juvenile crime

Obviously a number of the effects on Bradshaw's list will not affect small children directly, but could certainly have an effect upon the family as a whole. It also needs to be remembered that unemployment rates for black and ethnic minority people have always been higher than the unemployment rates for white people (Oppenheim, 1993), and even if they have qualifications, these people are still more likely to have difficulty in finding employment. There are more women than men who are in low-paid employment, particularly as low pay is associated with part-time employment.

The child care worker needs to be aware of these facts and of the necessity to treat those from poor families with respect and under-standing. Child care workers can ensure that children from these families are encouraged in order to build up their self-esteem and confidence so that they benefit as much as possible by attending a playgroup, nursery or school.

Homelessness

It has already been mentioned above that the loss of employment could also result in a family becoming homeless. In the 1980s there was a lot of government encouragement for people to buy their own homes, including those people living in local authority accommodation. Following this boom, the UK experienced a recession and many people lost their jobs as companies folded or cut back on the numbers of workers they were employing. People with mortgages found that they were unable to pay them, and the mortgage companies re-possessed their homes, leaving families homeless. When a family with young children becomes homeless the local authority has a duty to find them accommodation. For many families the first stage is to be placed in temporary accommodation which may be bed-and-breakfast accommodation. In 1990 the London Boroughs Association estimated that there were 9,000 or more children living in bed-and-breakfast accommodation in London (Kumar, 1993). Families were likely to stay in bed-and-breakfast for anything between 50–67 weeks whilst waiting for the local authority to find them a permanent home. Most com-monly, bed-and-breakfast accommodation is only provided for the mother and children; the father will have to find himself accommoda-tion elsewhere. This effectively splits up the family and may lead to a permanent family breakdown. Living in temporary accommodation can have serious effects upon the physical, emotional and mental health of all the family members.

A second option for families who may have lost their home is to move in with relatives. Whilst this may seem preferable to living in bed-and-breakfast accommodation it can lead to overcrowding, quarrels and stresses for the resident family and the incomers. There are no accurate figures for the numbers of families living in this situation, as they may not come to the attention of the local authority or social services. Lack of amenities and lack of privacy can lead to marital conflict and maternal depression. Child care workers need to remember that children living in temporary accommodation, in cramped conditions or high rise flats will need extra opportunities for boisterous physical play which will develop their large muscle co-ordination and help them release excess energy.

Family Violence

As families find themselves in stressful situations and unable to cope with their problems there is a greater likelihood of family violence. Resorting to alcohol or drugs to 'drown their sorrows' can lead to normally tolerant people becoming violent. There are many reasons why violence may occur in families, such as low tolerance levels, lack of parenting skills, and/or pressures from outside the family such as poverty, unemployment, poor housing etc. Children of such families are more often the victims of violence than the perpetrators.

Although children may live in a household where there is violence between the parents or other adults, violence might not be shown towards the children. However, research undertaken by the NSPCC has shown a correlation between child abuse and domestic violence: in 45% of child abuse cases the mother was also being abused (Calouste Gulbenkian, 1995). Violence may not just be physical, as the Women's Aid Federation of England (in Calouste Gulbenkian, 1995) states:

> Violence can also mean among other things: threats, deprivation of food, limiting contact with family or friends, constant criticism, being locked in the house, intimidation, threatening children to exert power and control over women, stealing money from women or depriving them of money.

Children living in these situations are caught between a conflict of both parents; this in turn causes stress-related illnesses, emotional confusion, acceptance of abuse as a 'norm' of family life, guilt, isolation, fear and the likelihood that they will become abusing adults. Child care workers need to be sensitive in their handling of these children and help them re-gain their self-esteem and confidence. It is important that the adults in child care and education establishments encourage a non-violent atmosphere by promoting co-operative games, negotiating skills, sharing activities and teaching children how they can help each other. The discouraging of aggressive games with guns and other weapons, stories about violence, and dealing promptly with children who bully or threaten others will also make the children feel that there is a safe, secure, non-violent atmosphere in the nursery.

Scenario 1.1

Julia is 3 years old and attends your playgroup for five morning sessions a week. You are aware that Julia, her mother and older brother are living in bed-and-breakfast accommodation. Draw up a programme of activities for Julia and explain how these will answer her particular needs which arise from her home situation.

PROMOTING EQUAL OPPORTUNITIES

One of the fundamental principles of the Children Act 1989 is that the welfare of the child is paramount and that all children's needs must be met regardless of the child's age, sex, religion, race or ability. In order for carers to meet these needs they must have knowledge and understanding of the principles relating to good practice.

Anti-discriminatory practice is putting equal opportunities into action and this requires the examination of one's own values and expectations and re-adjusting these in order to ensure that, as a child care worker, you give all children and their families equality of opportunity. Anti-discriminatory practice is not just related to race or colour but also refers to gender, lifestyles, class distinctions and ability/disability. There is good evidence that certain groups in society are discriminated against and therefore find it more difficult to get employment or decent housing; they find themselves living in areas that are poorly served for pre-school provision, health clinics or a good transport system.

Child care workers also need to be aware of the negative stereotypical images of ethnic minorities, women, people with disabilities and people who are poor, which are depicted in the media. It is very damaging for children's self-esteem to grow up surrounded by negative images, therefore it is important that resources used with children, such as videos, books, posters, toys and games are carefully scrutinized to ensure that they do not contain negative stereotypes. There are organizations such as the Working Group Against Racism in Children's Resources, Letterbox Library and Early Trainers Anti-racist Network which are able to provide checklists, book lists and lists of suppliers to help child care workers select appropriate materials. (See also the list of organizations at the end of this book for addresses.)

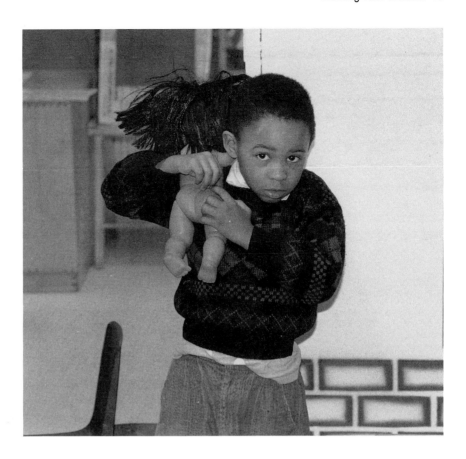

The Hidden Curriculum

This is the name given to the social roles, gender roles, attitudes and values that are communicated to the child in ways other than through the curriculum: the unspoken lessons that children learn from other children and adults.

From a very early age, children are absorbing information from what they see and hear around them; stereotyping and labelling can have a very damaging effect upon children. Making assumptions about children on the strength of how a previous member of the family behaved or how the child's parents behave, e.g. 'Well what can you expect of a child from that family, have you met the mother?', is very damaging to children and goes against good child care practice. Children that grow up feeling that they are inferior because of their colour, race, disability, or family background will not be able to reach their full potential.

> ### Scenario 1.2
>
> Sian has just married and now finds herself a step-mother to 4-year-old Sarah. Sian has no children of her own. Sarah has recently begun to exhibit behaviour problems at the nursery and at home. When Sarah is with Sian she has temper tantrums, is very demanding of sweets and toys, and is unco-operative and aggressive. What advice can you give to Sian to help her cope with Sarah?

Scapegoating and labelling

We live in a society that has a tendency to discriminate against certain groups: women, ethnic groups, people with disabilities, to name but a few. Blaming a particular group of people for our own misfortunes or things that are wrong in society is a form of scapegoating and is a very dangerous thing to do. Unfortunately, it is much easier to blame somebody else than to examine the situation and blame those who are really responsible, or undergo self-criticism in order to see where we have gone wrong. Most societies hold stereotypical views of one sort or another, for example, in Western society there is a stereotypical view that all scientists wear glasses and have white coats. How true is this? Researchers into this area have found that very few stereotypes are actually true representations. The media are responsible for creating and perpetuating many stereotypes within our society. Stereotypes often come to the fore when dealing with parents: how influential upon a carer's attitude towards a parent is what the person may be wearing, the spoken accent, whether they arrive in a car or walk?

Labelling is a form of stereotyping but usually refers to giving certain attributes to a child or person, the attributes being based upon stereotypes. A lot of labelling can take place in staff rooms where it may not be uncommon to hear remarks such as, 'We have Sally Y starting at playgroup today. I should watch out for her, I had her sister last year and she was a real problem.' Poor Sally has no opportunity to show that she is different from her sister; she has been labelled before she even enters the building.

Rosenthal and Jacobson (1968) carried out a very famous experiment called 'Pygmalion in the Classroom', where they told teachers the names of the children who would be high fliers and those who would not be so able. At the end of the experimental period all the children had lived up to their label as either high fliers or less able, in spite of the fact that Rosenthal and Jacobson's choice had been arbitrary and was not based on any prior knowledge of the children. This experiment shows just how powerful the labelling system is and how it is able to influence the teacher's expectations of the children. These findings were upheld by the Swann Report (1985) which found that teachers' low expectations were one of the main reasons for black children underachieving.

It is important that child care workers do not make assumptions about children or parents based upon dubious information. Many child care professionals have had the experience of thinking a child is the instigator of all the fights, only to find, when they have carefully observed the situation, that in fact the other children were provoking the child. This is one of the very important uses of child observation techniques. It is very daunting for a small child to have to prove that they are not as badly behaved as an older brother or sister, nor are they likely to behave in the same way as their outspoken, aggressive parent. We all know that some children relate better to some members of staff and this can result in two staff members giving conflicting reports on how a child behaves. It is important that children are accepted on their face value and treated accordingly.

Gender issues

It is not unusual in our society to find women/girls being treated differently from men/boys. This happens in the wider society and may be reflected within the home or in the playgroup or other pre-school facility that the child attends. The Sex Discrimination Acts 1975 and 1986 make it unlawful to discriminate against a person on the grounds of gender.

There is a large amount of research which shows that the early play experiences of girls are likely to result in them being less aware of space, less adept at large motor skills such as riding bicycles and using climbing frames. There is a tendency for child care workers to direct girls towards quiet activities, the home corner, the dressing up corner, the book corner etc. There is a tendency to direct boys towards the more boisterous activities such as bicycles, climbing frames, large building bricks, rough and tumble corners etc. If all children are to have equal access to all activities, with the staff giving all children equal encouragement to take part in these activities, then it must become a positive policy of the establishment rather than just left to the decision of each individual member of staff. The nursery or playgroup is the ideal place for children to experiment as it offers different experiences and opportunities which may not be available to them at home, for example boys being able to dress up or play with dolls.

Good practice in this area is reliant upon the attitudes of the staff and it is important that they do not discourage children from experimenting in this way. Staff need to be aware of the way in which they use

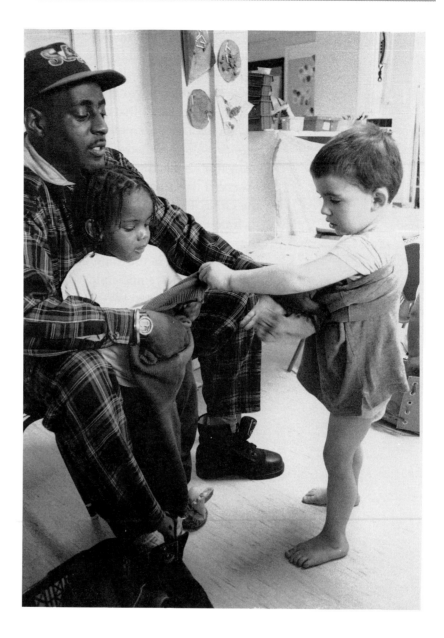

language which can reinforce gender stereotypes. Expressions such as: 'Boys do not cry', 'Girls should not climb trees', 'Boys do not dress up in girls' clothes', 'Girls do not play with trains', 'What a tom-boy you are Sarah', only succeed in deterring children from experimenting. Sexist attitudes can be as damaging to boys as they are to girls. Not all boys want to climb trees, play boisterous games or ride bicycles. When children are playing in the hospital corner it is most common to find that the boys are the doctors and the girls are nurses, but it is the duty of the carers to ensure that each child is given a turn at being a doctor or a nurse.

It is also important for the nursery or playgroup to exhibit positive role models which are not gender specific, for example, having books and stories about girls doing adventurous things and boys participating in caring activities, having pictures which show women driving buses, building houses, fighting fires etc. and men looking after children, preparing meals, nursing, caring for the elderly etc.

Race, colour and ethnicity

It has already been mentioned in this chapter that the UK is a pluralistic society. The population of the UK is made up of people from a wide variety of religious, racial and ethnic origins.

Immigration to the UK is not a new phenomenon; Peter Fryer (1984) records that the first black people arrived in Britain with the Roman army. In the 1800s there were large immigrations of Irish who were fleeing from the famine and Jews from Eastern Europe who were fleeing from the pogroms. The 1950s and 1960s saw immigrations of people from the West Indies, Asia and Africa. As the UK is a member of the European Union and there is now free movement between all 15 member states it is likely that there will be more French, Germans, Dutch, Danes etc. living and working in the UK. The UK has a Race Relations Act 1976 which, among other things, makes it unlawful to discriminate against people on grounds of race. However, laws do not stop people from treating other people differently; such changes require the individual to alter their attitudes.

All child care establishments should reflect the diversity of the society in their equipment, reading materials, pictures, displays stories, rhymes etc. The images around the nursery should be positive. If meals are served, menus should be varied in order to include foods such as pizzas, curries, tropical fruit, rice, stir-fry etc.

Staff need to be aware of the language they use and understand that the word 'black' is often used as a negative descriptor, i.e. blackleg, blackmail, black sheep.

Research by Milner (1983) and Maximé (1991) shows that children as young as 3 years of age understand the differences in colour and are aware of the racial hierarchy. Children learn this by seeing and hearing the people around them treating black people differently. This results in black children having poor self-esteem and gravitating towards a peer group where there are other black children. Siraj-Blatchford (1994) says that the most common form of racism experienced by young children is name calling or negative references to their colour or language. Sadly, research carried out by Wright (1992) found that it was not only the children who behaved in a racist manner but also the staff in the nursery and primary schools in her study.

Scenario 1.3

As a nursery officer you are concerned that the boys in your group of 4-year-olds are always playing violent games, shooting each other, mock fighting, bullying the smaller children and girls. How will you deal with this situation?

Disability

It is national policy wherever possible to integrate children with special needs within the mainstream facilities available for under-fives. The Education Acts (1981, 1988 and 1993) and the Code of Practice (1993) have made it easier to integrate such children into mainstream schooling. Some children may have special needs which require adaptations in order for them to access the nursery or school, such as a child with spina bifida who uses a wheelchair, whereas another child may have special needs which require extra staff time and attention, such as a child with a language deficit or behavioural problems. It is possible for any child to be categorized as special needs at some stage in their development, but with additional help they may be redesignated. For many children it is not always obvious to other children and adults that they may have a special need, such as those with sickle cell anaemia or cystic fibrosis, unlike those with conditions such as cerebral palsy or Down's syndrome.

Children with special needs are categorized as 'children in need' under the Children Act 1989. There has been controversy over this categorization as parents and experts argue that just because a child has a special need, it does not automatically mean that the child has needs that are not being met. However, the categorization does enable local authorities to give extra help and support to families that have pre-school children with special needs. This would enable the children to have a place in a nursery, nursery school or other pre-school provision which is supplied and paid for by the local authority. It also enables the local authority to arrange any necessary home adaptations which may be required or provide special equipment.

Children are always curious about each other and will ask questions about those children who appear to be different. Children's questions should be answered honestly and the positive images of the child with disabilities must be promoted by the child care worker. Sadly, Micheline Mason (1993) says

> We live in a system with a very rigid definition of who is valuable and who isn't... The expectations [*by society and individuals*] of

disabled people are lower than those of non-disabled people. Disabled children live in a system which has set up expectations of where the majority of young disabled people will eventually end up. Most people still expect disabled people to remain segregated for most of their lives.

If Mason is right then child care workers need to closely examine their expectations, values and attitudes in relation to children with disabilities. If children with disabilities are to be truly integrated into mainstream provision then this must take into account the importance of mainstream provision being able to offer an anti-biased equal opportunity environment. There must be positive role models and images of children and adults with disabilities; there must be stories that depict children with disabilities in 'heroic' positions. Children with disabilities must be encouraged to participate in all the activities in the nursery, playgroup or school. Staff must be careful not to be over-protective and should encourage children with disabilities to make decisions for themselves.

THE ANTI-BIAS CURRICULUM AND GOOD PRACTICE

Providing an anti-bias curriculum will not in itself eliminate discrimination within a child care establishment. However, Siraj-Blatchford (1994) states that by removing the biases which are harmful or counter-productive, this aids the well being of the children and their families and is a positive start. Staff need to take a pro-active approach, by listening to children, intervening when name calling or stereotyped ideas are being expressed and generally making it clear to children and parents that there are specific expressions and behaviours which are not acceptable within the nursery. All children need to feel equally valued and this can only be done by the worker considering the whole child, the whole curriculum and the whole environment. Staff need to look at themselves as individuals and as child care workers and examine the values and beliefs that they are transmitting to the children in their care.

Resources do not combat bias but they are tools to be used with the children and should therefore be carefully chosen to ensure that they reflect the anti-bias ethos of the establishment. Staff support and training may be necessary before an establishment can begin to look at its practice and devise a strategy for the future. Staff should work as a cohesive team, all working to the same anti-bias goals and able to share their experiences and use the expertise and advice of professionals. Equal opportunity policies are now common in most child

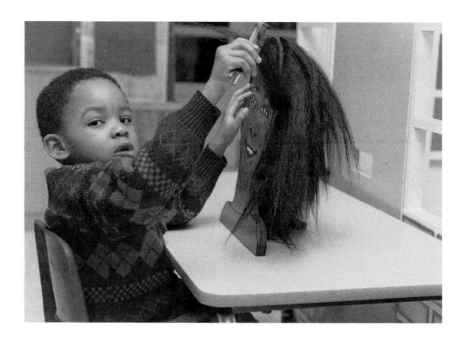

care establishments but in themselves do not lead to good practice. Any policy needs to be discussed and written by the whole staff team so that there is ownership and commitment to its implementation. A policy is no good if it is not translated into the everyday practices of the workers. Along with policies there is a need to develop strategies: how will the staff deal with racist, sexist or other derogatory remarks that are made by the children? How will staff respond to children who refuse to sit next to a black child or a child that has disabilities or a child from a poor family who may not be wearing designer trainers? How will the staff ensure that all children are being valued as individuals? Derman-Sparks (1989) offers a checklist that staff can use to monitor their own good practice; the following is an adaptation of this:

◆ Do child care workers pick up on non-verbal and verbal expressions of interest as quickly with girls as they do with boys? With differently abled children? With black children?
◆ Do child care workers offer girls as much physical freedom and use of large motor equipment as they offer boys? Do they allow boys freedom to express feelings? Do they help more often or do more for girls than boys?
◆ Do child care workers provide adapted opportunities for children with certain limitations to interact actively and independently with

materials and other children? Do they over-help or over-protect children who are different?

◆ Are similar behaviours interpreted and responded to differently with boys than with girls? White children than black children? Able bodied than differently abled children? For example do child care workers respond differently to an aggressive act of a boy or a black child or a child with special needs?

Scenario 1.4

The staff at your community nursery have decided to develop an anti-bias curriculum. As the senior worker it is your task to explain what this means to the Management Committee and to ask them to release the appropriate resources in order to put the idea into practice. Draw up a presentation for the Management Committee which clearly states the underlying principles of the anti-bias curriculum, the strategies for implementation and the resources that will be required.

Finally, Iram Siraj-Blatchford (1994) offers the following list that child care workers can use to ensure that they are offering an anti-racist curriculum:

The curriculum will:
◆ develop an understanding that people come from a range of backgrounds and cultures and offer children a secure environment in which to explore their own culture;
◆ offer opportunities for children to explore that no culture, language or religion is more superior than others;
◆ depict a range of families;
◆ show people from a range of ethnic backgrounds doing everyday things;
◆ use the children's interests in planning, and to extend their learning;
◆ find appropriate resources and examples from a range of cultures for each topic over and above the everyday multicultural toys, poster etc;
◆ depict a range of child rearing practices from different cultures;
◆ help children talk about and challenge stereotyping;
◆ promote social and emotional development...;
◆ involve parents and community groups...;

◆ illustrate through the curriculum that human achievements are universal and not just western;

◆ expect high standards of achievement from all the children.

Assignments

1. Write an essay on the advantages and disadvantages of living in an extended family.

2. What effects does poverty have on the lives of family members?

3. What do you understand by bed-and-breakfast accommodation? What are the possible effects that bed-and-breakfast accommodation could have on a child's development?

4. 'Poverty is a phenomenon of the lower social classes'. Discuss this statement.

5. What do you understand by the term 'low pay'? What type of families are likely to find themselves in a low pay situation? What government benefits are low pay families able to claim?

6. You overhear Raymond (aged 5 years) calling Peter (aged 4 years) a 'spastic'. What action, if any, do you take?

7. You overhear a member of staff telling Sally (aged 4 years) that girls do not climb trees. What action, if any, do you take?

8. What do you understand by the term 'hidden curriculum'?

REFERENCES AND FURTHER READING

Andreski, Ruth and Nicholls, Sarah (1995). *Setting Standards: a guide for the nursery professional*. Nursery World, London.

Aspinwall, Kath (1984). *What are little girls made of? What are little boys made of?* NNEB, St Albans.

Bradshaw, Jonathan (1990). *Child Poverty and Deprivation in the UK*. National Children's Bureau, London.

Braun, Dorit (1992). Working with parents. In *Contemporary Issues in the Early Years* (ed. Gillian Pugh). Paul Chapman/NCB, London.

Browne, Naima (1993). Girls and boys go out to play. *Childcare Now*, **13**(1), p. 20.

Browne, Naima and France, Pauline (1986). *Untying the Apron Strings: anti-sexist provision for the under fives*. Open University Press, Milton Keynes.

Burgoyne, Jacqueline and Clark, David (1982). Reconstituted Families. In *Families in Britain* (ed. Rapoport RN, Fogarty MP and Rapoport R). Routledge & Kegan Paul, London

Calouste Gulbenkian Foundation (1995). *Children and Violence: Report of the Commission on Children and Violence.* Caloustc Gulbenkian Foundation, London.

Candappa, Mano (1995). Equal opportunities and ethnicity in early childhood services. *Childcare Now,* **15**(3), p. 10.

Cochran, Moncrieff, Larner, Mary, Riley, David, Gunnarsson, Lars and Henderson, Charles (1993). *Extending Families: the social networks of parents and their children.* Cambridge University Press, Cambridge.

Commission for Racial Equality (1996) *From Cradle to School.* A practical guide to racial equality in early childhood education and care, revised edition. Commission for Racial Equality, London.

Derman-Sparks, Louise (1989). *Anti-bias Curriculum: tools for empowering young children.* National Association for the Education of Young Children, p. 8., NAEYC, Washington DC.

Derman-Sparks, Louise (1993). How to challenge bias in childcare. *Co-ordinate,* no. 33, January, p. 8. VOLCUF, London.

Dixon, Bob (1990). *Playing Them False: a study of children's toys, games and puzzles.* Trentham Books, Staffordshire.

Drummond, Mary Jane (1993). Learning about Gender Bias. *Co-ordinate,* no. 33, January, p. 17.

Elfer, Peter (1995). *With Equal Concern...* National Children's Bureau, London.

Equal Opportunities Commission (1995). *An Equal Start. Guidelines on equal treatment for the under eights.* Equal Opportunities, Wales, Cardiff.

Fryer, Peter (1984). *Staying Power: the history of black people in Britain.* Pluto Press, London.

Grabrucker, Marianne (1988). *There's a Good Girl: gender stereotyping in the first three years of life.* Women's Press, London.

Kenway, Penny and Hyder, Tina (1995). Offering children an equal start. *Co-ordinate,* no. 45, January, p. 4.

Kumar, Vinod (1993). *Poverty and Inequality in the UK: the effect on children.* National Children's Bureau, London

Lane, Jane (1995). No equality no quality. *Childcare Now,* **15**(3), p. 8.

Leach, Penelope (1994). *Children First.* Michael Joseph, London

Mason, Micheline (1993). Disability bias. pp. 13-14. *Co-ordinate,* no. 33, pp. 13-14.

Maximé, Jocelyn E (1991). Towards a transcultural approach to working with under sevens. In *Report of Two Conferences Combating Racism among Students, Staff and Children.* NCB/EYARN.

Milner, David (1983). *Children and Race: 10 Years on.* Ward Lock Educational, London

Moss, Peter (1988). *Childcare and Equality of Opportunity.* European Commission, Brussels.

Newsom, John and Newsom, Elizabeth (1976) *Seven Years Old in the Home Environment.* London: Allen & Unwin.

Oppenheim, Cary (1993) *Poverty the Facts.* Child Poverty Action Group, London.

Phillips, Angela (1993) *The Trouble with Boys: parenting the men of the future.* Pandora, London.

Potts, Patricia (1993) Learning for all. *Child Care Now,* **13**(1), p. 9. Day Care Trust.

Pre-school Playgroup Association (1991) *Equal Chances: Eliminating Discrimination and Ensuring Equality of Opportunity in Playgroups.* PPA, London.

Reiser, Richard and Mason, Micheline (1990) *Disability Equality in the Classroom: A Human Rights Issue.* Inner London Education Authority. (Available from: Disability Equality in Education, 78 Mildmay Grove, London, N1 4PJ.)

Robson, Brenda (1989) *Pre-school Provision for Children with Special Needs.* Cassells, London

Rosenthal, R and Jacobson, L (1968). *Pygmalion in the Classroom.* Rosehart & Winston, New York

Siencyn, Siân Wyn (1993) Bilingual start for young Welsh. *Childcare Now,* **13**(1), p. 19.

Siraj-Blatchford, Iram (1994) *The Early Years: laying the foundations for racial equality.* Trentham Books, London.

Slaby, Ronald, Roedell, Wendy, Arezzo, Diana and Hendrix, Kate (1995) *Early Violence Prevention: Tools for Teachers of Young Children.* National Association for the Education of Young Children, Washington DC (available in UK from Early Years Training Network (formerly VOLCUF)).

Sudbury, Julia (1993) Challenging racism in the early years. *Childcare Now,* **13**(1), p. 15.

Swann Report (1985) *Education for All.* HMSO, London.

Tizard, Barbara, Blatchford, Peter, Burke, Jessica, Farquhor, Clare and Plewis Ian (1988) *Young Children at School in the Inner City.* Lawrence Erlbaum Associates, London.

Troyna, Barry and Hatcher, Richard (1992) *Racism in Children's Lives.* Routledge/NCB, London.

Twitchin, John (1988) *The Black and White Media Show Book. Handbook for the study of racism and television.* Trentham Books, Staffordshire.

Wolfendale, Sheila and Wooster, Janine (1992) Meeting special needs in the early years. In *Contemporary Issues in the Early Years* (ed. Gillian Pugh). Paul Chapman/NCB.

Wright, Cecile (1992) Early education: multicultural primary school classrooms. In *Racism and Education* (ed. D Gill). Sage, London.

Young, Michael and Willmott, Peter (1962). *Family and Kinship in East London.* Penguin Books, Harmondsworth, Middlesex.

Chapter 2

Child Health

This chapter covers underpinning knowledge for all or parts of the following unit for the National Vocational Qualifications (NVQs) in Child Care and Education: C2
Also linked to CACHE awards modules: Diploma Modules E, D, M; Certificate Modules 4.

INTRODUCTION

If children are to be kept safe from disease and illness it is important that the child care worker has a good grasp of the underlying principles of health. The child care worker has a responsibility to ensure that the children in his/her care are able to enjoy their developmental experiences and activities without being exposed to undue risks in the environment. Part of this responsibility involves the child care worker carrying out measures in order to prevent primary infection or the spread of disease to the children in their care.

In the Victorian era, diseases such as tuberculosis were common and quickly spread through a population which had poor diet, poor washing facilities, poorly heated accommodation and dubious personal hygiene. Present day living conditions and our greater knowledge of how diseases are spread goes a long way to preventing the outbreak of epidemics within society.

The World Health Organization (WHO) defines the following factors as essential to the health and development of children:

◆ Food and drink in sufficient quantity and nutritionally adequate
◆ Warmth
◆ Fresh air
◆ Exercise
◆ Rest and sleep
◆ Good posture
◆ Personal and communal health
◆ Dental care
◆ Sensible clothing
◆ Prevention of illness and injury
◆ Medical supervision

The responsibility for ensuring that children receive the above basic needs rests with the government, individual families and carers.

MULTI-CULTURAL ASPECTS OF CHILDREN'S ILLNESSES

Throughout this chapter there will be descriptions of signs and symptoms of common childhood ailments. It must be noted that these descriptions only apply to white skin. In children that have brown or black skin tones, rashes will look different from the descriptions given here; for example, on a black skin a rash will not look red, although it will still be raised or have vesicles. It should also be noted that where reference is made to skin pallor again this refers to white skin. Children with black or brown skin do go pale when they are sick, however, this is not always as obvious as it is in white skin, in fact the child may look greyish. Parents and carers who are familiar with the child will be able to recognize skin pallor in a black child but it may not be so obvious to others. If a black child is having difficulty in breathing any blueness of the skin may be difficult to detect, therefore there is a need to check the child's lips and fingernails. If these are showing signs of blueness then this will denote cyanosis which indicates a serious breathing problem requiring immediate emergency treatment.

INFECTIONS

All disease is caused by germs, which is a generic term to describe three types of infection: bacterial, fungal and viral (Table 2.1). Once germs have established themselves in a favourable situation they have a very fast breeding rate, some doubling their numbers every half hour. The period when the organisms are multiplying but the body is not showing any symptoms of the disease is the incubation period.

Table 2.1 Common infectious diseases of childhood

Disease: Common cold (Coryza)
Incubation period: 1–3 days
Cause: Virus
Method of spread: Airborne, but can also be spread by hands through infected person touching eyes, mouth and nose, and hence carrying pathogens in secretions
Signs and symptoms: Sneezing, sore throat, stuffy nose, running nose; headache, partial deafness; slight rise in temperature (pyrexia), child irritable, not interested in play
Complications: Sinusitis, laryngitis, tracheitis, bronchitis
Treatment: No specific cure; symptoms treated; comfort and hot drinks; junior paracetamol if prescribed by doctor; vaseline applied to nostrils to prevent soreness due to discharge

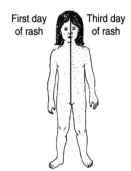

First day of rash   Third day of rash

Disease: Measles (less common since vaccinations became available)
Incubation period: 1–2 weeks
Cause: Virus
Method of spread: Airborne
Signs and symptoms: Running nose, watery eyes, fever, cough; Koplik's spots – red with white centres – may be seen inside the mouth in 1 or 2 days then disappear; 3rd day fever subsides; 4th day temperature rises again maybe as high as 104°F as rash appears; blotchy red rash spreads down over the body from the face; child fretful, irritable, hot, with cough and painful eyes
Complications: Otitis media (middle ear infection), pneumonia, corneal ulceration (rare), encephalitis (rare)
Treatment: Requires special attention. Drugs may be prescribed to prevent complications; relief of symptoms; bedroom/sickroom shaded if photophobia (sensitive to light) present; attention to diet as vomiting may occur; plenty of fluids; convalescence in fresh air and sunshine

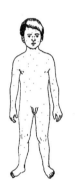

Disease: Chickenpox (*Varicella*)
Incubation period: 2 weeks
Cause: Virus
Method of spread: Airborne (and by discharge from skin lesions)
Signs and symptoms: Mild onset – off colour, slight pyrexia; rash appears first on trunk, then face, then limbs; lesions are little vesicles (blisters) surrounded by a ring of inflammation; blisters can erupt easily; vesicles become filled with pus (pustules) then dry up to form scrabs; rash appears in crops so three stages vesicles, pustules and scabs may all be seen at one time; child will feel ill, with severe headache and find spots irritating
Complications: Scarring and secondary infection only if there is scratching of spots
Treatment: Calamine lotion is soothing for irritation; relief of other symptoms; particular care of skin to prevent chafing and complications; child's nails should be cut short to prevent secondary infection through scratching, gloves applied if itching is severe; if lesions are profuse penicillin may be prescribed to prevent secondary infection

Disease: Mumps (epidemic parotitis)
Incubation period: 2–3 weeks
Cause: Virus
Method of spread: Airborne
Signs and symptoms: General malaise, pain and swelling of parotid glands (in front of and under the ear) on one or both sides of the face; rise in temperature, sore throat, headache may develop before glands swell; flow of saliva may increase or diminish – affects feeding; jaws painful – patient may refuse feed or find difficulty in chewing
Complications: Meningitis (rare), orchitis (inflammation of testes, usually only in adolescent boys) rarely causes sterility

Table 2.1 (continued)

Treatment: No specific cure; care of mouth – cleanliness and moistness; plenty of fluids, through a straw (which has a good effect on the child who may be feeling miserable and will enjoy departure from normal methods of drinking)

Disease: Whooping cough (pertussis)
Incubation period: 1–2 weeks
Cause: Bacillus
Method of spread: Airborne
Signs and symptoms: Affects mainly children under five; cough usually first sympton often accompanied by clear, watery, nasal discharge. Coughing becomes more frequent then paroxysmal and temperature rises; whoop follows a number of short, sharp, expiratory coughs; the cough reflex closes the glottis and the child cannot take a breath until the outburst is over: thus he appears to be suffocating – may turn blue, red or purple, eyes seem enlarged and protruding; drawing in air against the resistance of the glottis causes whoop. Production of thick mucus and vomiting usually follows the cough; paroxysms of coughing may leave the child exhausted; babies do not usually acquire whooping cough
Complications: Otitis media, bronchopneumonia, convulsions in babies under 1 year old – may lead to brain damage
Treatment: Requires extra special attention. Coughing may continue for several weeks; the child may be reluctant to have feed because of vomiting; paroxysms are less frequent after 2–3 weeks and temperature is usually normal in about 2 months. Child must be kept warm, moist inhalations can be given and linctus may be prescribed for the cough; antibiotics may be prescribed to prevent complications in the chest. Support and comfort should be given during paroxysms which are frightening; a feed may be given after an attack to give time for absorption before the next coughing fit

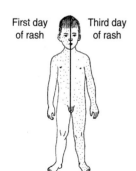

First day of rash   Third day of rash

Disease: Rubella (German measles)
Incubation period: 2–3 weeks
Cause: Virus
Method of spread: Airborne
Signs and symptoms: Mild symptoms – headache, stiff neck, running nose, rash of pink spots behind the ears and forehead, may be swollen glands at back of neck; child may feel unwell
Complications: Only if contracted by women in first 3 months of pregnancy – baby may be born with deafness, heart abnormalities and general malformations
Treatment: Treat symptoms

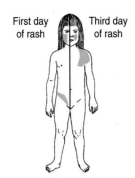

First day
of rash

Third day
of rash

Disease: Scarlet fever (scarlatina)
Incubation period: 2–7 days
Notifiable disease
Cause: Bacillus
Method of spread: Droplet infection
Signs and symptoms: Sore throat, swollen lymph glands in the neck, tonsils may be covered with purulent discharge, bright red rash appears on second day lasting 2–3 days, with flaking of skin over area of rash, especially on palms and soles of feet
Complications: Uncommon
Treatment: Isolation, antibiotics, treat symptoms

Disease: Dysentery (means inflammation of colon and rectum; can be caused by amoebae or bacilli, but bacillary type most common in UK)
Incubation period: 1–7 days (usually 3–4 days)
Cause: Bacillus
Method of spread: Excreted in stools so spread through poor sanitation, poor sewage disposal and by lack of hand-washing. Spread in food
Signs and symptoms: Diarrhoea often with blood and mucus; fever, headache, muscular pain; diagnosis made by taking specimen of stools, or from a rectal swab
Complications: Shock and prostration, dehydration through loss of fluid and salts; can be fatal, particularly in young children and babies
Treatment: Isolation; excreta disposed of only after disinfecting; fluid or low-residue diet, i.e. foods which are easily digested such as fruit purees, jellies, thickened soups, eggs, minced meat and fish, ice-cream. Drugs as prescribed by the doctor. Three negative swabs required before patient is pronounced cured. Strict hygiene in food handling. Important that child is given plenty of fluids

Disease: Gastroenteritis (infantile)
Cause: *Escherichia coli*, *Salmonella* or dysentery bacillus, viral infection or secondary to other infection, e.g. otitis media
Method of spread: Rare in breast-fed babies
Signs and symptoms: Looser bowel action sometimes with blood or mucus or coloured green or bright orange; occasional vomiting and rejection of feeds despite obvious thirst and hunger. Reduced urinary output, weight loss, dehydration; restlessness and general malaise
Complications: Dehydration often rapid and severe with metabolic and electrolyte disturbances; these, if uncorrected can lead to convulsions, renal failure and death
Treatment: Requires special attention. Give child plenty of fluids such as plain cooled boiled water.

Bacteria

These are micro-organisms which are made up of a single cell. They are not all harmful to the body, in fact a number of bacteria live in the gut and aid the digestive processes. Harmful bacteria produce toxins which are not able to be neutralized by the body's natural defence mechanisms (called antibodies) and this results in illness. Bacterial infections can be treated with antibiotics, although overuse of antibiotics has led to some bacteria becoming resistant to them. Examples of harmful bacteria are *Streptococcus*, which causes sore throats, scarlet fever; *Staphylococcus*, which causes boils, styes etc; *Diplococcus*, which causes pneumonia, meningitis (bacterial type) etc.; bacilli, which cause tuberculosis, typhoid etc.

Fungi

These are plants which do not have chlorophyll and feed on dead or living organic matter. They are the same family as mushrooms, toadstools, moulds and lichens. Those that live on or in the human body are much smaller and often cannot be seen without a microscope. The most common illnesses caused by fungal infections are thrush and athlete's foot. Fungal infections are easily treated with anti-fungal medications. They do not require treatment with antibiotics.

Viruses

These are very very small micro-organisms which operate in a complex way by invading the cells of the body and altering the way that the cell behaves. They cause illnesses such as mumps, measles, influenza, polio etc. In general they are not treatable with antibiotics, but the body is able to build its resistance to common viral infections by immunization.

Scenario 2.1

Mary is a childminder and one of the children that she cares for is Donna aged 2 years. Today Donna seems unwell, she has a rise in her temperature, a runny nose, watery eyes and looks generally unwell. When Mary examines her she looks in her mouth and finds that Donna has small white spots like breadcrumbs inside her mouth. What do you think is wrong with Donna? What action will Mary need to take?

SPREAD OF INFECTION

There are four main routes by which infection is able to enter the body:

1. *Inhalation* – the organism is breathed out by an infectious person and then inhaled by the next person who will then become

infected. Examples of illnesses passed on in this way are the viral diseases influenza and measles.

2. *Ingestion* – the person becomes infected by eating contaminated food or drinking contaminated water. Illnesses spread in this way are, e.g. salmonella poisoning, typhoid.

3. *Inoculation* – the organism gains access to the body through a wound in the skin, or the bite of an insect. Illnesses spread in this way are, e.g. malaria and post-operative wound infections.

4. Very rarely, infection can be transmitted before a child is born, via the placenta or the mother's blood supply. Examples of such illnesses are syphilis, AIDS/HIV.

People come into contact with infection through a number of ways:

1. *Carriers* – people who have no symptoms of the disease but who are still able to pass the disease on to other people. They may be people who have had the disease and are now in the convalescent stage. A person is unaware that they are the 'carrier' of a disease. The most famous 'carrier' was a woman known as 'Typhoid Annie' who was thought to have been responsible for a widespread typhoid epidemic which took place in the United States during the last century.

   Another type of carrier is called a vector. This is when an organism passes on a parasite, for example the Mosquito transmits the malaria parasite. Household pets such as cats, dogs and birds act as vectors and can pass worms and fleas on to children.

2. *Direct spread* – through bodily contact with the infected person. Illnesses which are passed on by direct contact are referred to as being contagious. Examples of these are impetigo and some forms of conjunctivitis.

3. *Indirect spread* – through the handling of infected objects such as dressings or contaminated faeces. In other cases contaminated food or water may lead to the indirect spread of diseases such as salmonella poisoning, typhoid and cholera. The contamination may have reached the food via flies, which are known to be responsible for the spread of dysentery, gastroenteritis, influenza and poliomyelitis.

4. *Airborne or droplet spread* – minute droplets from the nose and mouth of an infected person are spread by sneezing, or dry out and are then spread by the air. Illnesses spread in this way are the common cold, respiratory tract infections, measles, mumps, chickenpox and other common childhood illnesses.

THE BODY'S DEFENCES TO INFECTION

The body has a number of ways of defending itself against infection. Externally, the skin has a protective function, as do the tear ducts in eyes and the mucous membrane in the nose. The nasal passages also have tiny hairs (cilia) which line the nose and act as filter mechanisms for germs.

Internally, the body has a lymphatic system which consists of a series of lymph glands connected by lymphatic vessels (tubes). The lymph nodes (glands) produce lymphocytes which are capable of destroying foreign antigens and of producing antibodies. These are part of the body's immune response to infection. Lymph nodes also act as filters for infection; the tonsils are lymph nodes.

The white blood cells (leucocytes and phagocytes) fight infection by producing an immune response in the body. When infection is present the number of leucocytes present in the blood is increased.

Antibodies are proteins formed in the spleen or lymph nodes which are produced as a response to the antigens of invading bacteria. Antibodies can be produced by a person actually having the illness and therefore becoming immune to contracting the same disease again, for example, measles. They can also be triggered off by the introduction into the body of antigens; this is how a number of immunization vaccines work. Thus the measles vaccine will introduce a mild form of measles antigen into the body which will then produce antibodies to offer the person immunity against measles; this is called acquired immunity.

Antitoxins are a type of antibody which neutralizes toxins that are formed in the blood by certain types of bacteria. As with antibodies, they can be produced by a person having the illness or they can be artificially introduced by the injection of a weak strain of the toxin, as in the case of tetanus.

TYPES OF IMMUNITY

Immunity is the power of resisting infection due to the effects of antibodies and antitoxins. There are two types of immunity, active and passive.

Active Immunity

This is the way the body responds to the antigens and toxins produced by bacteria or other types of infection. There are two types of active immunity, natural and artificial.

Natural active immunity

This is when immunity has been acquired through:

1. Actually having an attack of the disease and producing antibodies which give lifelong immunity, e.g. measles, rubella

2. Having a mild attack of the illness which may show very few symptoms but which docs invade the body's defences enough to produce antibodies. Repeated mild attacks of an illness will produce the same effects

Artificial active immunity

This is when immunity is acquired through inoculation with:

1. Living organisms, e.g. smallpox vaccine
2. Living weakened organisms, e.g. BCG (Bacillus Calmette–Guerin), tuberculosis vaccine
3. Dead organisms, e.g. whooping cough (pertussis) vaccine
4. Modified toxins (toxoid), e.g. diphtheria vaccine

Passive Immunity

This may be acquired naturally or artificially.

Natural passive immunity

This is the immunity which a baby obtains from its mother. Part of this immunity would have been passed to the child whilst it was still in the womb, via the placenta. Additional immunity is passed to the child via the mother's milk; this is why breast feeding is so important, particularly in those early days following the birth.

Artificial passive immunity

This offers temporary protection from a disease by injecting serum from a person or animal. The effects will only last 3-4 weeks, as once the antibodies die out, so will the immunity. It is not used very often as it only has a short term effect.

IMMUNIZATION

Before the discovery of vaccines, many children died from the common childhood illnesses such as diphtheria, whooping cough (pertussis), smallpox. Even today, in countries where there is no comprehensive child immunization programme, children still die or are left permanently damaged due to contracting common childhood illnesses.

Although there has been negative publicity given on the side effects of some types of immunization, particularly the link between whooping cough (pertussis) vaccine and brain damage, the dangers of the diseases are much greater than the small risks associated with children being immunized.

The reasons for immunizing children are:

◆ Some infectious diseases are extremely dangerous and can be fatal in children under 1 year, e.g. whooping cough (pertussis)

♦ Complications of infectious diseases may cause handicaps or disability, e.g. poliomyelitis can cause permanent paralysis, measles can affect eyesight and hearing

♦ Complications from infectious diseases can also affect the child's intellectual development, e.g. convulsions leading to brain damage (a complication of whooping cough (pertussis))

♦ Immunization reduces the number of people who will contract the disease and eventually this can eliminate the disease within society, e.g. the World Health Organization (WHO) now classes smallpox as having been eradicated

Table 2.2 Immunization schedule[a]

Immunization	Age
Triple vaccine (DTP)[b] and polio	2 months (1st) 3 months (2nd) 4 months (3rd)
Measles, mumps, rubella (MMR)	12–18 months[c]
Booster (DT and polio)	4–5 years
Rubella (girls only)	10–14 years
BCG (tuberculosis – tuberculin-negative children)	10–14 years[d] or infancy
Booster (tetanus and polio)	15–18 years

[a] Based on recommendations from a pamphlet issued by the Department of Health (1990)
[b] Diphtheria, tetanus and pertussis (whooping cough)
[c] May be given at any age over 12 months
[d] Interval of 3 weeks between BCG and rubella

PREVENTION OF THE SPREAD OF INFECTION

Diet, fresh air and exercise all go towards preventing the spread of infection. In addition to these there are a number of practices which the child care worker needs to carry out as a matter of routine when dealing with children and these can be found in the following hygiene procedures put forward by the Department of Health (1992), which, although written for those who deal with HIV positive children, are good practice for all situations.

Hygiene Procedures
1. The following hygiene procedures are recommended as safe practice for all staff and all those who care for children whether in private homes or group settings. The procedures should not be

limited to those knowingly involved in the care of children with HIV. These are common sense precautions which will protect against a range of minor and major infections which may be transmitted via blood and body fluids...

General Measures

2. Cuts or sores which break the skin on the hands should be kept covered with waterproof adhesive or other suitable dressing.

3. Hands should be washed thoroughly:
- before and after carrying out First Aid procedures involving external bleeding and/or broken skin
- after contact with blood or body fluids (semen, faeces, urine or vomit

4. Where possible, disposable gloves should be used when carrying out First Aid. Household rubber gloves should always be used if heavily soiled material, or bleach, is being handled. It is important to ensure the safe storage of bleach in areas which involve children and to which children have access.

5. Razor blades, toothbrushes etc. which may be contaminated with blood should not be shared. (Needles etc. used for intravenous therapy at home should be stored/disposed of in appropriate containers supplied by the Health Service. The same safety precautions will apply to injecting equipment used for any other purposes, e.g. where someone has an injecting drug habit. They should be encouraged to take all the necessary safety precautions to prevent 'sharp' injuries to others including children.)

Accidents Involving Blood

6. Normal First Aid procedures should be followed, and should include the use of disposable gloves where possible. The wound should be washed immediately, squeezing to expel blood and using plenty of soap and water, and a suitable dressing applied or pressure pad if needed. Medical advice should be sought as soon as possible.

7. If blood is splashed onto the skin it should be washed off immediately with soap and water. Splashes of blood into the eyes or mouth should be washed out immediately with plenty of water.

8. After accidents resulting in bleeding, surfaces with blood on them, e.g. tables or furniture, should be cleaned liberally with household bleach, freshly diluted 1 in 10, that is 1 volume (e.g. cupful) of bleach should be added to 9 volumes (cupfuls) of water to make the required (effective) 1 in 10 solution. Alternatively, hot

soapy water may be used. Bleach can corrode metal and burn holes in fabrics if used for too long or in the wrong concentration, and must never be used on the skin.

Cleaning

9. Normal cleaning methods should be used. No special disinfectants are necessary for either bath or toilet. Disposable cloths should be used, with a separate one for the kitchen, for the bathroom and for the toilet.

10. Spillage of blood, vomit and body fluids should be cleaned up as soon as possible. Ordinary domestic bleach, diluted 1 part in 10 parts with water, or hot soapy water, should be poured gently over the spill which has been covered with paper towels. If possible and if this is convenient the diluted bleach should be left for 30 minutes. It should then be wiped up with disposable paper towels. More solid spillages, such as vomit or faeces, can be scooped up in a bucket of hot soapy water and the scoop cleaned or disposed of as contaminated waste.

11. Paper towels should be treated as infected waste. Disposable gloves and aprons should be thrown away as infected waste.

12. Clothing and linen (e.g. terry nappies, sheets, towels) which have been soiled with blood or body fluids should be washed in a well maintained washing machine, rinsing initially in the cold rinse cycle and then washing in the hot wash cycle (approximately 80 degrees centigrade). Overloading should be avoided. If handwashing is unavoidable, household rubber gloves must be worn and the water and detergent must be as hot as can be tolerated and the articles rinsed in hot water.

13. Crockery and cutlery can be cleaned by handwashing with hot soapy water or in a dishwasher or dish sterilizer.

Disposal of Waste

14. Items which have been soiled with blood or body fluids may be flushed down the toilet if disposable (e.g. tampons) or burnt (e.g. paper towels, disposable nappies, sanitary towels). If this cannot be done on site, the rubbish, including protective disposable gloves or aprons, should be 'double bagged' in plastic bags and effectively secured. Arrangements should be made with the local authority for collection of this infected waste for incineration. Vomit, urine and faeces should be flushed down the toilet and potties should be washed with detergent or antiseptic and hot water and dried with paper towels.

(Department of Health, 1992)

In addition to the Department of Health recommendations the following practices should also be carried out as part of the basic routine:

◆ Always wash your hands before handling food
◆ Always wash your hands after using the toilet or helping a child to use the toilet
◆ Always wash your hands before touching a baby or making up a baby's feed
◆ Ensure that bathrooms, toilets and baby changing areas are cleaned/disinfected frequently and at least daily
◆ Report to the parent or officer in charge any child with abnormal stools, high temperature or other sign of infection
◆ Only use disposable handkerchiefs and ensure that, once used, they are kept away from the reach of children
◆ Encourage and teach children to wash their hands after using the toilet and before meals
◆ Be familiar with the establishment's policy for dealing with diarrhoea and other gastrointestinal infections
◆ Ensure that each child has their own flannel, towel, toothbrush and hair brush, and that these are washed/disinfected frequently
◆ Any cuts or open wounds on the hands should always be covered when dealing with children or food, or rubber gloves should be worn
◆ Toys and other playthings should be washed/disinfected regularly, particularly soft toys

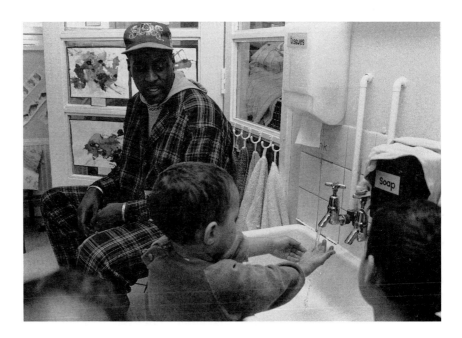

- Ensure that children always wash their hands after playing with pets and do not let animals lick children's faces or hands
- Ensure that all pets are free from worms or fleas and that hutches and tanks etc. are cleaned regularly

SIGNS OF ILLNESS IN CHILDREN

How do you know when a child is feeling ill? There are a number of physical and behavioural signs that will alert the adult to sickness in a child. The child may feel hot, look flushed and have a raised temperature. There may be vomiting, diarrhoea or both. The child may complain of pain or that a part of them is hurting. They may become breathless or have difficulty in breathing. They may lose their appetite and refuse to eat or drink. They may look pale, with dark rings around their eyes. They may have constipation or difficulty in passing urine. They may have a rash or some other type of skin irritation. In addition to the physical signs there may also be changes in their behaviour. They may be fretful and crying or may become listless and withdrawn. They may cling to their parent or carer, not wanting to leave them or join in activities with the other children. They may be sleepy and not want to wake up after their afternoon nap. They may regress and forget their toilet training or only want to play with toys suitable for a younger age group. They may just generally not seem to be their normal selves.

DEALING WITH A SICK CHILD

If you are responsible for a child that becomes sick there are a number of important steps to take. First you need to ascertain whether the situation is an immediate emergency, for example, any difficulty in breathing, loss of consciousness or a convulsion would require immediate medical treatment. It is important to inform your superiors and/or the child's parents about the situation. The child should be made comfortable, resting in a quiet place with their favourite toy. The child will need to be reassured as they may be very frightened. You should make a note of any symptoms to give to the parents/doctor. If the child is vomiting or has diarrhoea, try to give them sips of water. Do not give any medicines unless they have been prescribed by a doctor. If the child has a very high temperature you should try to bring this down by tepid sponging and putting an electric fan in the room. A sick child should not be left alone.

COMMON CHILDHOOD ILLNESSES

This section looks at illnesses that are likely to be encountered by the child care worker. There is not room in this book to cite every likely illness that affects children; however, what is given is a selection of the most common. Some of the illnesses cited are minor and others are more serious and have long lasting effects on the child's lifestyle. The illnesses are in alphabetical order to make it simpler for the reader to find a reference quickly.

Asthma

This is a respiratory disease characterized by recurrent attacks of difficulty in breathing, usually accompanied by wheezing and coughing. It is due to an obstruction in the airway caused by a spasm of the muscle fibres in the walls of the bronchioles (the small air passages in the lungs). The spasm reduces the size of the airway and this restricts the flow of air. Asthma can occur at any age but is most common in children. It can occur anytime following birth but the higher incidence appears in children age 3 years and upwards. Childhood asthma sometimes disappears during the teenage years. Asthma does have an hereditary factor, often running in families and is more commonly found in males. In recent years there has been a marked increase in the incidence of childhood asthma although the reasons for this are unknown. Four main causes of asthma have been identified:

1. Direct irritation of the bronchiole membrane by dust, chemicals, air pollutants
2. Reflex irritation of the bronchiole membrane from infection elsewhere, i.e. sore throat, nasal infection, gastric infection
3. Allergy to pollen, animal fur, feather pillows, house dust, certain foods etc. In these cases the child may also suffer from eczema or other forms of dermatitis
4. Psychological factors such as fear, anxiety and severe emotional trauma may trigger an attack

An acute asthma attack can be a very frightening thing for the child, parents or carer. The most important thing is to stay calm and reassure the child; if the child gets nervous or begins to panic it will make the attack far worse. If this is a first attack the doctor should be called immediately. It is important that the urgency of the situation is clearly relayed to the doctor. If the attack gets worse and the child is having great difficulty breathing and their colour is poor (blue around the lips and mouth, looks pale) then an ambulance should be sent for, ensuring that the emergency telephone operator is made aware that the patient is a child with serious breathing difficulties. An acute asthma attack will usually respond to the administration of drugs such as ephedrine, adrenaline, antihistamines etc.

Once the child has recovered from the acute attack phase the asthma is likely to be controlled with inhalers or other medicine.

Doctors also may recommend a sensitivity test in order to try to determine whether the cause is an allergic reaction.

Coeliac Disease

This is an inherited disease whereby the lining of the intestine is damaged by gluten, a protein found in wheat, rye, barley and some other cereals. The condition usually appears between the age of 6–24 months. The child will fail to thrive, will lose their appetite and have diarrhoea with bulky offensive stools. Diagnosis is made by taking a biopsy of a piece of the lining of the intestines. Once the diagnosis is made the disease is treated by giving a gluten free diet; this means eating only cereals where the gluten has been removed. Children with the condition will need to stay on this diet for the rest of their lives.

Conjunctivitis

This is an inflammation of the conjunctiva (membrane which covers the front of the eye). The eye may have a sticky discharge and the conjunctiva, which is normally colourless may appear pink; there may also be irritation as if a piece of grit had got into the eye. There are a number of bacteria and viruses which can cause conjunctivitis and it is also a complication of measles. It is easily remedied by getting prescription eye drops from the doctor. It is important to try to prevent the child rubbing the eye as the infection is easily spread to both eyes and to other children or family members.

Convulsions

A convulsion is a violent uncontrolled movement of muscles in the body which may be accompanied by loss of consciousness. A convulsion is always a serious sign and will always require medical attention. Febrile convulsions occur in some children when the child has a high temperature. They are most common in children between the age of 1–3 years and usually do not occur in children over the age of 5 years. The doctor should be called immediately and whilst waiting for the doctor the parent or carer should try to bring the child's temperature down by tepid (not cold) sponging, cooling with an electric fan, opening windows, removing excessive clothing and bedcovers.

Cystic Fibrosis

This is an inherited disease occurring in about one in 2000 births. Approximately one in 20 adults are carriers of the gene; where two carriers have a child there is a one in four chance of it having cystic fibrosis (this particular ratio is known as a Mendelian recessive). The gene is mainly found in people of Indo-European origin.

The condition affects all the mucus-secreting glands in the body whereby they do not secrete runny, watery discharge but thick viscous discharge which blocks the connecting tubes. It may be diagnosed in the first weeks of life due to failure to thrive, as the lack of pancreatic juices prevents the digestion of food; there is also diarrhoea with offensive faeces due to the inability to digest fat and a cough due to chest infection. However, more commonly the diagnosis is made in the first few years of life with the child having repeated chest infections and the inability to digest foods. The diagnosis may be confirmed by examination of the child's faeces and their sweat which will have a high sodium chloride content.

The long term management of the disease is by giving pancreatic enzymes, vitamin supplements and a low fat, high sodium chloride diet. Daily physiotherapy is carried out by the parents/carers in order to clear the mucus from the lungs.

Diabetes Mellitus

This is caused by the pancreas failing to secrete enough insulin, which prevents the body storing and using glucose. The glucose remains in the blood, and sugar is secreted in the urine. The incidence of diabetes in the population is increasing and is now at a level of about 1.5% of the population diagnosed as having the disease. Diabetes in the under-five age group is rare but one-fifth of all diagnosed diabetics are children.

The first signs of diabetes are a sudden intense thirst accompanied by excessive urine output. If this stage goes undetected by parents/carers then the child is likely to become lethargic, drowsy and may go into a coma. It is easy to diagnose by urine and blood tests. Diabetes can be controlled by giving daily insulin injections in conjunction with a low carbohydrate diet. The amount of insulin given needs to be finely balanced as too much insulin can lead to the child going into a coma (hypoglycaemia) and too little can also lead to a coma (hyperglycaemia). Hypoglycaemia can happen very quickly and as it is the result of having too little sugar in the blood, sugar lumps or high glucose drink will reverse the situation. Children often become familiar with the early warning signs of hypoglycaemia and should carry glucose tablets or sugar lumps in their pockets. If the child becomes unconscious before they can be given sugar/glucose then an ambulance must be called as they will require emergency treatment.

If the child has been eating foods which are not on their diet programme they may have too much sugar in their blood for the insulin to be able to neutralize; this will lead to a hyperglycaemic coma. The child must be seen immediately by a doctor and if the child is unconscious then an ambulance should be called. If the reason has been that the child has eaten too many sweets or other tempting goodies which they are not allowed it is no use being cross with the child. It must be explained to the child that they do have an illness and how important it is for them to help control the illness by not eating forbidden foods. Although certain precautions need to be taken with diabetic children they should lead a normal lifestyle participating in all activities.

Scenario 2.2

Samantha is a nanny caring for Jamie aged 18 months. Jamie has recently had a bad cold, with a raised temperature and has been sleeping a lot. Samantha goes to his bedroom to wake him after a nap and finds that he is twitching and writhing about in an uncontrolled fashion. What do you think is happening to Jamie? What action must Samantha take?

Diarrhoea

This term refers to frequent bowel motions which pass loose, fluid faeces. For children the most dangerous side effect of diarrhoea is dehydration (sudden loss of fluid in the body) and can lead to death if it goes untreated. Diarrhoea in babies/young children is often accompanied by vomiting (gastroenteritis) which is far more dangerous than diarrhoea alone. Babies who are bottle-fed are very susceptible to gastroenteritis, which they can contract through infected feeding bottles. Bottle-fed babies sometimes have diarrhoea due to too much sugar in the feed or the fat content of the milk being too high.

There are numerous causes of diarrhoea, such as infection, food poisoning, high temperature, or an allergy to cow's milk or a certain food. It can also be a symptom of another illness, e.g. coeliac disease or cystic fibrosis.

All cases of diarrhoea should be taken seriously, and if prolonged over a period of 24 hours in children over 2 years then medical advice should be sought. For children under 2 years medical advice should be sought at the onset. If it is accompanied by vomiting then medical advice should be sought immediately.

Eczema (Dermatitis)

Another name for eczema is dermatitis and both are generic terms for a number of different skin diseases. Eczema is an inflammation of the skin and is very common as one in eight children may suffer from this at some time in their lives. A common cause is thought to be external irritants which trigger the body's immune system to respond. Dermatologists are of the opinion that those people who suffer from eczema or other forms of dermatitis have a particularly sensitive immune system, and it is thought that the trait is inherited and is passed through families. It is not uncommon to find children who have eczema also suffering from more than one allergic illness, for example asthma or hayfever. Children may have a mild form of eczema or a severe form and it can last for a few months or over a number of years.

The doctor will be able to offer a number of remedies depending upon the type of rash and the severity of the rash (Table 2.3). It is also useful to try to avoid substances which may cause irritation to the skin, for example by using pure cotton garments next to the child's skin rather than wool or synthetic fibres. It is also better to use bath oils in place of soap and use non-biological washing powders for the child's clothes. Putting cotton gloves on the child at night can prevent damage through scratching.

Table 2.3 Characteristics of eczema rash[a]

Characteristic	Description
Itching	This is the worst aspect because it can be so upsetting for the child. It also makes them scratch, which can lead to more rawness, soreness and infection
Redness	This is caused by extra blood flowing through the blood vessels in the skin in the infected area
A bubbly, grainy appearance on the skin	These are tiny fluid-filled blisters just under the skin called 'vesicles'
Weeping	This happens when the blisters burst, either by themselves or because of scratching, and the fluid oozes out onto the surface of the skin
Crusts	These are scabs which form when the fluid dries
Scaliness	Children with eczema often have a dry, scaly skin. This may be a result of the disease but may also be the natural skin type of that family which, in some people, can predispose them towards developing eczema
Pigmentation	Pale patches of skin can appear because eczema can disturb the production of pigment which controls skin colour. The effect does fade and disappear
Lichenification	This means a leathery, thicker skin area in response to scratching. Again it does fade

[a] Source: Hilton (1993)

Seborrhoeic dermatitis (cradle cap)

This type of dermatitis is not related to eczema or other types of dermatitis. Cradle cap occurs in young babies and is caused by the glands on the scalp producing too much sebum (grease). It appears as brown scaly patches which may cover the whole scalp. There is no need for medical treatment as the condition disappears of its own accord. Baby oil can be used to soften the crust. The health visitor will also be able to advise on the best type of shampoo to use when a baby has cradle cap.

Failure to Thrive (FTT)

This is not actually an illness but a cluster of symptoms which may be associated with some of the illnesses mentioned in this section. There appears to be no agreed definition of FTT but it is generally used to describe infants/children who fail to gain weight. It results from the failure to obtain or use the necessary calories required for growth. Betz *et al.* (1994) describe three categories of FTT (see also Table 2.4):

Organic FTT is caused by physical factors such as congenital heart defects, gastro-intestinal disorders, renal disease, central nervous system abnormalities, chronic infections, endocrine disorders.

Non-Organic FTT is an absence of any (medical) history, physical or laboratory findings that indicate organic disease capable of causing FTT. It is caused by environmental factors that affect the child's intake or use of calories. The problem is usually due to a complex set of interactive patterns between the infant and the care givers.

Mixed FTT is caused by a combination of organic and non-organic factors. For example, a child with a cleft lip is unable to suck adequately because of the physical deformity (organic cause). The inability to suck, in turn, can interfere with the mother's feelings of adequacy. She may then stimulate and caress the infant less. The interplay of positive messages and reciprocal play associated with feeding is, therefore, blocked to a degree.

There is a view that non-organic FTT is a symptom of child neglect caused by maternal deprivation. However, this is not the accepted view of all paediatricians as some advocate that whatever the cause it is a genuine clinical illness.

Table 2.4 Indicators of potential failure to thrive

Physical Indicators

Weight below the 3rd percentile[a]

Sudden or rapid deceleration in the growth rate

Delay in developmental milestones

Muscular hypotonia

Decreased muscle mass

Generalized weakness

Abdominal distension

Behavioural Indicators

Avoiding eye contact

Intense watchfulness

Avoidance of physical contact with other people

Repetitive self-stimulating behaviours (e.g., rocking, head banging, head rolling, and intense sucking)

Disturbed affect (e.g., excessive irritability, apathy, or extreme compliance)

Sleep disturbances

Lack of age-appropriate stranger anxiety

Inappropriate lack of preference for parents

[a]Measurement relates to standard height/weight charts for normal development

Glue ear

This is a very common condition affecting 17/20 children under the age of 6 years. Modern hearing tests and diagnostic procedures have led to an increase in diagnosis of this condition. Glue ear is the name given to the condition whereby the fluid in the middle ear becomes viscous and glue-like, blocking the eustachian tube and, if left untreated, is likely to damage a child's hearing. It is easily treated by inserting 'grommets' (tiny hollow tubes of plastic) into the ear drum to equalize the pressure within the ear drum and aid the draining of the fluid. 'Grommets' are inserted under a general anaesthetic so the child may have to stay in hospital overnight or attend a special day surgery unit at the hospital.

Haemophilia

This is a sex-linked inherited disease which affects the clotting ability of blood. It affects males but is passed on through the female genes as the defect is on the sex-linked chromosome (there is a rare form of haemophilia which is not sex-linked and therefore affects both males and females and this is called Von Willebrand's disease). In haemophilia the blood is unable to clot due to a lack of the anti-haemophilic factor, commonly known as Factor 8. A child with haemophilia will get spontaneous bruising which is the result of bleeding into the skin tissues; there is also bleeding into the joints, such as knees, ankles and elbows, which make them appear red and swollen. Haemophiliac children need to be protected from boisterous play which may lead to injury or bleeding. Because of the spontaneous bruising, child care workers and health visitors may mistake an undiagnosed haemophiliac child as a victim of child abuse. It is therefore always wise to refer any cases of bruising in children to the paediatrician or GP to avoid misdiagnosis.

Haemophiliacs can be treated by transfusions of blood products which contain Factor 8. Sadly, some haemophiliacs were given Factor 8 from the USA which was contaminated with the HIV virus. From 1985 onwards all blood was carefully tested for HIV/AIDS and therefore this situation should not recur. Some of the haemophiliacs who were infected with the HIV virus have subsequently developed AIDS (Acquired Immune Deficiency Syndrome).

Scenario 2.3

You are in charge of a mixed age range group of children in a family centre. Beth aged 3 years is a new child and she is diagnosed as having cystic fibrosis. What information will you need to obtain from Beth's parents? Write a programme for Beth's daily routine. What, if any, special precautions will you need to take for Beth?

Headlice

These are parasites which live on hairs and feed by sucking the blood of the host. They are about 1–4 mm long, greyish white in colour and multiply at a very fast rate. They are very easily spread when children put their heads together or swop hats or hair ribbons etc. Headlice used to be viewed as a result of poor hygiene and children with headlice were stigmatized by being sent to special clinics; they were made to sit away from the other children and had to play alone. Fortunately, the progress of science has shown us how headlice are spread and how infestation is not necessarily associated with poor living conditions or neglect.

The first sign that a child may have headlice is that the parent or carer notices the child scratching their head due to irritation caused by the bites. A careful examination of the hair may reveal small white dots on the hairs, particularly behind the ears and at the nape of the neck. The white dots are the eggs of the lice (nits) which are fixed to the hair by a cement-like substance, so that unlike dandruff they do not flake off. The mature headlouse lays about 60 or more eggs a month and these take 7 days to hatch and are fully grown in about 2 weeks. Treatment is by the application of a special shampoo or lotion such as Prioderm which can be purchased from the chemists or obtained free from local health clinics. It is important to follow the instructions when applying the shampoo or lotion and the child's hair must be left to dry naturally as any applied heat, such as that from a hair dryer, will stop the chemicals taking effect.

If a child at nursery or school has become infested with headlice it is important that the staff take precautions to prevent the spread. All hats in the dressing-up corner should be removed and thoroughly washed in disinfectant. Each child should have their own comb and brush as a matter of routine good practice and these should be regularly washed and disinfected. Children's hats and coats should be kept on their own pegs and children should be discouraged from trying on each others hats, slides, ribbons etc.

Hepatitis

This is the name given to inflammation of the liver which in children is likely to be caused by a virus. There are two types of hepatitis virus, A and B. Most cases of hepatitis in the UK are caused by virus A whereas hepatitis contracted abroad is most likely to be virus B. There are vaccinations against both types of hepatitis virus. Symptoms of hepatitis are loss of appetite, headache, fever and jaundice (where the skin and whites of the eyes become yellow). Hepatitis is very infectious and therefore strict hygiene precautions must be used when dealing with infected children. There is no specific treatment except rest and a high protein diet.

HIV/AIDS

HIV (Human Immunodeficiency Virus) is the virus that is thought to cause AIDS (Acquired Immune Deficiency Syndrome), although not all HIV positive people develop AIDS. There is no test for AIDS; all that the scientists know at present is that people that have AIDS also test positive for HIV and that some people who are HIV positive have developed AIDS. The virus was first identified in the 1980s, although it is now known that there were cases of AIDS before this date but they went undiagnosed.

HIV is known to be transmitted in the following body fluids:

◆ Semen
◆ Vaginal and cervical secretions
◆ Blood
◆ Blood products, i.e. plasma, clotting factors

Although HIV has been found in other body fluids such as saliva, urine, breast milk, tears and amniotic fluid, there is no evidence to show that it has ever been transmitted through these routes. The most common routes for transmission are through unprotected penetrative intercourse, and the sharing of syringes and needles by drug abusers.

There are three routes by which children may become infected with HIV:

1. Being a haemophiliac and becoming infected by being given infected blood products (see under haemophilia)
2. Having acquired the virus from their mothers
3. By being sexually abused by a person who is HIV positive. In these circumstances the transmission is the same as for the adult population

Most of the children in the UK who are HIV positive have acquired it via their mothers, who are likely to have been drug abusers. Before birth the virus may be transmitted across the placenta to the developing foetus, during birth the virus may be transmitted via blood or vaginal and cervical secretions and after birth it may possibly be transmitted in the breast milk.

Between 10% and 20% of HIV positive women will pass the virus to their baby. Doctors are unsure about breast milk being a route by which HIV is passed to children; however, HIV positive mothers are recommended not to breast-feed their babies.

All babies whose mothers are HIV positive will have the mother's antibodies in their blood. These antibodies do not disappear until the child is around 2 years of age; it is therefore difficult to diagnose children under 2 years as definitively being HIV positive.

For the child care worker there is a greater risk of prejudice against children who are HIV positive than of them developing the disease; it is therefore important that the child care worker maintains a high level of confidentiality to avoid the child and family being stigmatized. As the Lambeth Women and Children's Health Project (1992) points out,

> There is no known case anywhere in the world of HIV infection having been transmitted in child care settings or schools.

There are other infections such as hepatitis which are much more common than HIV and transmitted much more easily. There is therefore no reason why an HIV positive child should not be treated the same as all other children. Good hygiene practices should be followed at all times to protect workers and other children against infection (see

Department of Health Guidelines in 'Prevention of the Spread of Infection' above). It is very possible that a child care worker may not know which children are HIV positive; this will depend upon the confidentiality policy of the establishment or local authority. Under the Children Act 1989, HIV positive children will come into the category of 'children in need' and this means that the local authority has a duty to ensure that help is provided for the families in order to enable them to meet the needs of the child.

Impetigo

This is a staphylococcal or streptococcal infection of the skin. It may develop as a complication of another skin complaint such as eczema or scabies. Impetigo starts with red spots which develop into blisters and these burst and form brownish crusts. It usually affects the scalp, face or hands. It is highly contagious (spread through touching) and extra care must be taken to prevent the spread of the infection to other children or carers. The doctor is able to prescribe antibiotics in the form of cream or tablets.

Nappy Rash

This is a rash that appears in the nappy area causing discomfort and pain for the baby. It can be caused by leaving the baby in a wet nappy and rubber pants for too long, as a reaction to detergents or biological soap powders, not properly drying the nappy area following a bath, or by the spread of seborrhoeic dermatitis from the baby's scalp (see under *eczema*).

It is treated by carefully cleaning the nappy area and then applying cream such as zinc and castor oil to the affected area to act as a waterproof barrier. The rash will heal more quickly if the baby can be left without a nappy for a few hours per day. Rubber pants should not be used and all nappies should be sterilized and washed in a detergent which is non-biological or specifically for baby clothes or children with allergies.

A more severe form of nappy rash can be caused by urine which is strong in ammonia. This type of rash is rarely seen in breast-fed babies as the strong ammonia in the urine is caused by a bacteria which thrives in the conditions produced by cow's milk feeds.

Scenario 2.4

Jenny works in a playgroup as a volunteer. Jenny notices that a number of children in her group are frequently scratching their heads. What do you think is wrong with the children? What action will Jenny need to take? What should she say to the children's parents?

Rickets

This is a disease of the bones which is caused by lack of vitamin D. It used to be very common in the UK until the 1940s when the government started the fortification of margarine with vitamin D. With the introduction of better diets and free school milk the disease was virtually eradicated. However, the Rickets Report (Sheiham and Quick, 1982) showed that there has been a significant increase in rickets and osteomalacia, particularly amongst Asian groups. Rickets is the name given to the disease when it occurs in children whose bones are still forming, and in adults it is called osteomalacia. Vitamin D is obtained from dietary sources or through the action of sunlight on the skin. Vitamin D is found in foods such as oily fish, liver, eggs etc. The prevalence of rickets and osteomalacia amongst the Asian community is mainly a result of their migration to the UK. People who have been used to living in the Asian sub-continent would have relied upon the sunshine to supply them with vitamin D and would not have needed to be concerned that they were getting this in their daily diet. However, following immigration to the UK they did not have the amount of sunshine they needed in order to keep up levels of vitamin D, and their diets may have changed very little from what they ate in Asia. Asians who have been born in the UK are likely to have a more varied dietary intake through school meals and eating in fast food establishments and restaurants; and through school nutrition projects and other health education programmes they are likely to be aware of the need for a diet rich in vitamin D. It is most likely that there is now less of an increase in rickets in the UK than there was in the 1980s, but there may still be an increase in osteomalacia amongst the older Asians.

Rickets leads to deformities of the bone such as bow legs or knock knees, and arm, skull and rib deformities. Osteomalacia leads to aching bones, listlessness and weakness of muscles in adults and fragile brittle bones in the elderly.

Ringworm (Tinea)

This is not a worm but a fungus which invades the skin, hair and nails. The fungus spreads down hair follicles and causes ring-shaped scaly patches. Ringworm is highly contagious and is easily spread to the other children or carers. It is easily treated with Griseofulvin ointment. Another type of infection caused by a similar fungus is athlete's foot which causes itching between the toes, this is most often transmitted in swimming baths and school shower rooms or other communal changing rooms.

Sickle Cell Disease

This is a term used to cover a number of blood diseases which are the result of an inherited disorder of the haemoglobin in the red cells. The red blood cells become sickle shaped, hence the name of the illness. It is found in people who themselves or their ancestors have come from African countries. Those with the sickle cell gene were protected from certain forms of malaria, thus it became a favoured gene in countries where there was malaria. In the UK the gene is carried by Africans, Afro-Caribbeans, people from the Middle East, South Asia and the Mediterranean. Mares *et al.* (1985) estimated that one in 400 of the UK's African and Afro-Caribbean population had sickle cell disease and one in 10 were carriers of the gene. In order for a child to inherit the disease they must have two parents who have the gene. With both parents carrying the gene the child will have a one in four chance of inheriting the disease. If only one parent has the gene then the child will have a 50/50 chance of being a carrier of the disease. Carriers of the disease are described as having sickle cell trait.

The first symptoms of sickle cell do not usually appear until the child is 3–6 years of age. The sickle shaped cells only live for 10–20 days, unlike normal red blood cells which live for approximately 120 days. The constant breakdown of the sickle cells causes chronic anaemia. The shape of the cells makes it difficult for them to pass along small blood vessels and they can become clumped together and stop the blood supply; this often occurs in the hands and feet. When this happens the child will have a lot of pain and this is described as a sickle cell crisis. A crisis can also be brought on by dehydration, strenuous exercise and infection. The constant breaking down of the red cells also leads to enlargement of the spleen. Sickle cell is diagnosed by a blood test. There is no routine screening in the UK for those children who are thought to be at risk from the disease, unlike the USA where a 1972 Act of Congress ensures that there are services for voluntary screening and diagnosis, counselling, education, medical referral and research. Sickle cell disease is not always easy to diagnose as the symptoms may be slight and may only be discovered during a routine blood test before an anaesthetic or during pregnancy.

There is no cure for sickle cell disease and the treatment is one that aims to relieve the symptoms. There is a good prognosis for sickle cell sufferers, and as medical science makes progress so they are able to have a longer and longer life span.

Parents and/or carers of a child with sickle cell disease will need clear and practical information on how to manage the child's condition. There is a Sickle Cell Society (details can be found at the back of this book) which is able to offer information and support to both sufferers, families and those who are working with people that have the disease. As with any genetic disease, parents will often feel very guilty, as they are responsible for their child's condition. It is therefore important that child care workers appreciate this and treat the parents with a high level of understanding and sensitivity.

Thalassaemia

Like sickle cell disease, thalassaemia is an inherited blood disorder. It mainly occurs in people from the Mediterranean areas such as Spain, Cyprus, Portugal, Italy etc., but there are also people with this 'gene who come from North Africa and India. It is inherited in the same ratios as sickle cell disease; those with the disease are described as having thalassaemia major and those who are carriers are described as having thalassaemia minor.

In thalassaemia the red blood cells are unable to produce haemoglobin which operates efficiently as it is unable to utilize iron. It can be diagnosed during the first 6 months of life as these children have severe anaemia and show symptoms of failing to thrive. It is treated by giving blood transfusions, and bone marrow transplants have proved successful. They also need regular injections of a drug which will counteract the excessive amounts of iron in their bloodstream. There is a good prognosis for thalassaemia sufferers, although there is no cure for the condition.

REST AND SLEEP

In order for children to stay healthy they need an adequate amount of rest and sleep. Sleep enhances tissue restoration and enables the body to relax, which promotes alertness during the waking hours. Children who are tired are more susceptible to infections and tend to be bad tempered and fretful. New babies will soon establish a pattern between waking and sleeping, and as they get older they will sleep for fewer hours. No two children are alike in their sleep patterns and some children may need less sleep than others. Children, like adults, will develop their own individual sleep patterns. Adults need to encourage children from an early age to develop different sleeping patterns for night and day. This can be done by giving the baby a great deal of stimulation during its daytime waking periods and trying not to give any stimulation during night-time waking periods.

Although children need a comfortable place to sleep, this does not necessarily mean their own bed; sleeping arrangements will differ between families and cultures. In some cultures it is traditional for small children, even babies, to sleep in the same bed as their parents. There used to be a fear that in taking a baby into bed with adults put it at risk of being suffocated by the adult rolling on top of the baby. Dr Hugh Jolly (1985) points out that slow motion films of babies in bed with their parents have shown that a normal baby will wriggle its way into a position so that it can breathe easily and that parents have a tendency to roll away from the baby. The only rider to this is that the adults must not be under the influence of alcohol or sleeping pills, as this dulls their normal reactions which would safeguard the baby. In the UK it is common practice that most children have their own cot/bed which is surrounded by their favourite toys, although this may be in the bedroom of the parents or the room of a sibling.

Most parents look forward to the day when their baby will sleep throughout the night; however some children may do this at an early

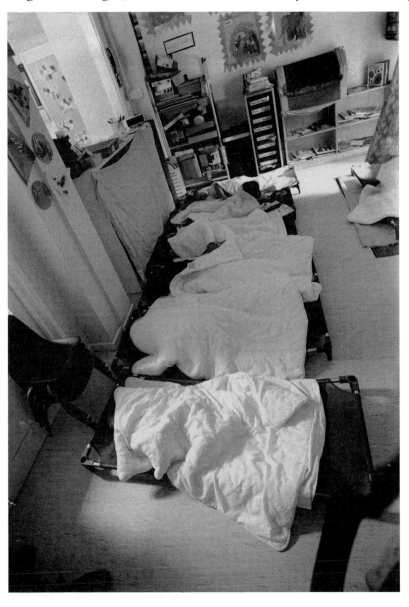

age, whereas others might take longer. It is important to develop a bedtime routine with children. This usually starts with bath time, saying goodnight to the family and being read a story once they are tucked up in bed with their favourite toy.

As they increase their waking hours, most children will need a nap during the day. In the early days this will be mid-morning and another mid-afternoon. Once children are old enough to go to play-group or part-time nursery school, it is easier if they have their nap during the part of the day that they are at home. Most playgroups and nursery schools do not have facilities for children to have a nap. If a child is in a day care situation then the child care worker will need to talk to the parent about the child's sleeping habits. They will need to find out when the child likes to go to sleep, what favourite toy or comforter they like to have with them when they sleep, whether they have a story before sleeping and how long they are likely to sleep for.

As children get older and become interested in television, it becomes more difficult to get them to bed at a reasonable time. Parents and carers must be firm about keeping to a specific bedtime as children that are tired during the day have difficulty concentrating and this inhibits their learning.

As children get older they may develop fears which either prevent them from sleeping or make them wake up during sleep. Children, like adults, will have dreams and nightmares, but they are too young to recognize these and talk about them. It is a good idea to leave a small electric night-light on in the child's room so that if they do wake they do not find themselves in complete darkness. Children who are frightened to go to sleep may be worried that their carer is going to leave them, so it always a good idea to put them to bed yourself and to reassure them that if they wake up you will be there.

EXERCISE

All children need exercise, room to move around and stretch their limbs, and time in the open air. Movement and exercise helps the child's physical development and gives them the opportunity to develop muscle co-ordination and gross motor movements. A period of time in the open air will stimulate the circulation of the blood, enable them to obtain vitamin D from the sunshine and improve their appetite. Most children are able to gain enough exercise by being given the opportunity to play indoors and outdoors.

Assignments

1. Visit your local infant welfare clinic and write a comprehensive account of what the clinic is able to offer parents and children.

2. Write an essay debating the advantages and disadvantages of immunizing children against whooping cough (pertussis).

3. Describe the special care that you would need to give to a 7-year-old child in your class who has been diagnosed as having sickle cell disease.

4. Write an account of how you would deal with a 4-year-old child who is having an asthma attack.

5. What do you understand by the term 'health screening'? Write an essay explaining what this is and its relevance to child health.

REFERENCES AND FURTHER READING

Betz, Cecily Lynn, Hunsberger, Mabel and Wright, Stephanie (1994). *Family-centred Nursing Care of Children,* 2nd edition. Philadelphia, W. B. Saunders.

Claxton, Rosie and Harrison, Tony (1991). *Caring for Children with HIV and AIDS*. Edward Arnold, London.

Department of Health (1992). *Children and HIV: guidance for local authorities.* HMSO, London.

Department of Health and Social Security (1980). *Rickets and Osteomalacia. Report on the Working Party on Fortification of Food with Vitamin D.* Committee on Medical Aspects of Food Policy. HMSO, London.

Griffiths, Ronno (ed.) (1992). *HIV/AIDS and the Under Fives. A guide for workers and carers.* Manchester AIDSline Women's Group: Manchester.

Hilton, Tessa (1993). *The Great Ormond Street Book of Baby and Child Care*. Bodley Head, London.

Jolly, Hugh (1985). *Book of Child Care*. Unwin: London.

Lambeth Women and Children's Health Project (1992). *HIV/AIDS: A Guide for Carers of Young Children.* Lambeth Women and Children's Health Project, London.

Leach, Penelope (1989). *Baby and Child: From birth to age five.* Penguin, London.

Mares, Penny, Henley, Alex and Baxter, Carol (1985). *Health Care in Multi-Racial Britain.* Health Education Council and National Extension College, Cambridge.

O'Hagan, Maureen, and Smith, Maureen (1993). *Special Issues in Child Care.* Baillière Tindall, London.

Sheiham, Helena and Quick, Alison (1982). *The Rickets Report.* Haringey Community Health Council, London.

VOLCUF (1991). *Keeping Children Healthy – a guide for under fives workers.* VOLCUF, London.

Chapter 3

Child Safety

This chapter covers underpinning knowledge for all or parts of the following unit from the National Vocational Qualifications (NVQs) in Child Care and Education: E2
Also linked to CACHE awards modules: Diploma Modules DGN; Certificate Modules

INTRODUCTION

It is a major responsibility of all child care workers to ensure that children are always in an environment which is safe. Accidents are the highest cause of deaths in children aged between 1–14 years. Under the registration procedures for the Children Act 1989 all premises where children are cared for must reach minimal levels of safety. It is the responsibility of the carer to ensure that these levels of safety are maintained from day to day and that they do not deteriorate following the visit of the registration officer.

A number of child care workers are nannies working in private houses who are not required to be registered under the Children Act 1989. For these people there is a responsibility to ensure that their employers are made aware of any areas in the house that may be unsafe and how these can be altered to make a child-safe environment.

Chapter 2 deals with safety in relation to infection and hygiene and this chapter concentrates on safety in the environment. In order for child care workers to be able to cope in the event of an accident they should hold a First Aid Certificate which is regularly updated.

FACTORS CONTRIBUTING TO ACCIDENTS

There are a number of factors which can contribute to accidents; these can be divided into *human factors* and *environmental factors*.

Human Factors

◆ Ignorance on the part of the carer about safety regulations. Ignorance is not a defence in a court of law; the person would still be held responsible as they have a duty to familiarize themselves with safety regulations
◆ Carelessness and lack of observation on the part of the carer. This

may be due to tiredness or fatigue or the carer having other things on their mind at the time

◆ Illness of the carer, which may affect their alertness to risky situations

◆ Influence of drugs or alcohol on the carer, which may make them careless or unaware of what is happening around them

◆ Not carrying out the routine safety regulations which have been explained to them or that they know that they should be taking

No carer should be left in sole charge of more children than they can be reasonably expected to control or keep safe. The Children Act Guidelines clearly state the ratio of adults to children in a variety of settings and these should be adhered to at all times. It is particularly important when a carer is taking children off the premises on a visit or outing.

Environmental Factors

◆ The siting of buildings and outdoor play areas can increase the risk of accidents

◆ Lack of gates or doors to prevent children wandering out of the room or building

◆ The internal arrangements in the home or nursery, particularly in relation to safety in kitchens, bathrooms, toilets and stairs

◆ Safety of furniture, play equipment, heaters, bedding, cots and windows

◆ Safe storage of sharp implements such as knives, scissors, cooking equipment

◆ Safety of clothing and footwear, particularly fire-retardant nightwear.

The following are just some of the ways in which child care workers can make the environment safe for children in their care. The Child Accident Prevention Trust and Royal Society for the Prevention of Accidents (addresses at the back of this book) are able to provide very full explanatory leaflets on safety. Unfortunately there is not enough space in this book to go into full details on accident prevention and the following represent just some of the precautions that can be taken.

ACCIDENT PREVENTION IN THE HOME

The Kitchen

All sharp implements should be kept in drawers or cupboards which have childproof fastenings (these are readily available in most DIY stores). All cookers should have a safety guard on the top to prevent children reaching up and pulling over saucepans (available from stores such as Mothercare and DIY stores). When the cooker is in use, all saucepan handles should be turned towards the back of the cooker so that they do not jut out across the top of the stove. Children should not be left alone in the kitchen. The doorway to the kitchen should have a gate to prevent children entering. All detergents, cleaning fluids etc. should be kept in a cupboard high enough to be beyond the reach of children. If such items are kept under the sink unit then the doors should have childproof latches. Fridges and freezers should have locks which need a key in order to open them. Tables should not have cloths as a child can topple a pot of tea or other hot drink by pulling the cloth. All electrical plugs should be of the safety childproof type. Any doors leading to the garden should have safety gates for use when the door may be left open, i.e. in the summer months. Kitchens should be equipped with a fire extinguisher and/or fire blanket.

The Lounge/Sitting Room

All furniture should be stable and not tip easily when a child leans on it. All electrical plugs should be of the child safety type to prevent children poking objects into the empty sockets. Coffee tables should be stable and should not have glass surfaces. Any ornaments or other precious artifacts should be kept on high shelves well away from the reach of children. Television sets, video machines and hi-fi equipment should be placed well out of reach of the children as should tapes, CDs and records. Video machines can now be purchased with a child lock in order to prevent children using adult or other unsuitable videos. Carpets should have non-slip surfaces and rugs should be backed with a non-slip substance. All fires or other exposed heating equipment should have a guard that is fixed to the wall. Windows should have child safety locks and bottom windows should not be opened when children are around, even in rooms on the ground floor. It is possible to get special safety devices which prevent windows being opened to a height which would enable a child to get through; these are available from good quality builders merchants or DIY stores. There should be no trailing flexes or other objects that could cause a child to fall. If furniture has rough corners these should have protectors, which can be obtained from children's equipment shops such as Mothercare.

The Bathroom/Toilet

All medicine cupboards should be situated well out of the reach of the child and have a lock. Cleaning fluids should be kept in a locked cupboard or on a shelf that cannot be reached by the child. When bathing children the cold water should always be put in before the hot water. The hot water temperature should be turned down so that it is not of a heat that would scald a small child were they to turn on the hot tap. Electrical equipment such as hair dryers should not be left in bathrooms. Bathrooms should not have open socket plugs but closed sealed electrical systems for heaters, razor points etc. (this applies even when there are not children in the household as it is a general safety rule). If the bathroom door has a lock this should be of the type that can be opened from the outside in the event of a child accidently locking themselves in.

The Bedroom

All bedding, pillows and mattresses should conform to the safety regulations for children's bedding. If they are purchased from a reputable shop they will be clearly marked with the safety kitemark. Cots must have bars that are close enough together to prevent the child's head being able to get through them and they must be painted with non-toxic paint. All toys should have the safety kitemark, particularly if they have eyes which might come loose. All children's nightwear should be fire retardant. Any open fires should be guarded with a fixed fireguard. Any windows should have safety locks and should only open at the top. Any furniture should be low enough to prevent children climbing up to the height of the window. All electrical plugs should be child safe and there should be no exposed or trailing wires.

The Garden

All gardening tools should be kept away from children, preferably in a locked garden shed. Any ponds or pools should be covered with strong wire to prevent children falling into them. Swimming pools should have special covers which can be purchased from pool suppliers. A special play area should be set aside for children where a swing or slide or other permanent fixed outdoor toy can be placed. It is best to fix such equipment in a grassed area so that if a child falls it is onto a soft surface rather than, e.g. concrete. Alternatively there are special rubber or woodchip surfaces which can be purchased specifically to act as a surface for outdoor equipment. Any plants which may be toxic to children (e.g. foxgloves, nightshade) should be removed from the garden. All weedkillers, fertilizers and other garden chemicals should be kept locked in the garden shed.

Scenario 3.1

Angela is a nanny who cares for Simon who is 18 months and Vanessa who is 3 years. Angela is visiting another nanny, Monica, who cares for Sarah aged 2 years. The children are playing in the sitting room with Angela and Monica. Suddenly Angela smells burning. What action should Angela and Monica take?

KEEPING BABIES SAFE

Babies are very vulnerable and will need special precautions for their safety during the first months of life. Babies need a safe place to sleep which:

◆ Is free of pillows, which can easily suffocate a baby
◆ Does not have fluffy blankets, particles of which can get into a baby's mouth and cause choking
◆ Is stable and not able to be tipped over if the baby moves around
◆ Does not have hanging mobiles that the baby can reach
◆ Does not contain toys with small parts that a baby could swallow
◆ Has high enough sides to prevent the baby rolling out of the bed

Babies are born with a very strong natural grasping reflex and they can quite easily pull pieces of material or other objects from toys or bedding. Avoid dressing children in lacy knitwear or clothing in which they can catch their fingers; ribbons around the neck can lead to choking.

A baby should not be left with a bottle propped in their mouth as this can lead to choking.

To help reduce the risk of cot death the Department of Health 1991 issued the following guidance:

◆ Lay babies on their back to sleep
◆ Do not over wrap or overheat them
◆ Do not expose them to cigarette smoke

Always keep small objects out of a baby's reach and if you leave them alone make sure the environment is safe. Always ensure that the baby has good support for head and back. At bath time put the cold water in the bath first and test the temperature before putting the baby into the water. Never leave a baby alone on a changing table.

SAFETY WHEN TAKING CHILDREN ON OUTINGS OR OUTSIDE THE HOME

Children should always be strapped securely into prams, pushchairs or buggies. When children begin to walk they should be kept on reins. If older children have a tendency to wander away from the carer, there is a restraining rein which can be purchased. The restraining rein is able to give the child a certain amount of freedom whilst at the same time ensuring that there is a link with the carer.

Children should be suitably dressed for the outing in clothes which protect them against the weather, hot, cold, wet or damp. Children should not wear their 'best' clothes and parents should be encouraged to dress them in casual clothes that do not require special cleaning or laundering. Children's clothing needs to allow them freedom of movement so that they can take full advantage of all the opportunities offered on the outing.

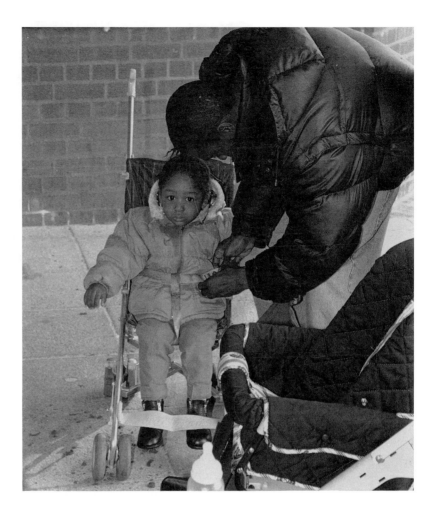

As soon as children are walking they should be introduced to road safety. At an early age, this is done by the example of the carer. Always cross roads at safe points such as traffic lights, zebra or pelican crossings. Always stop with the child at the kerb and check the flow of traffic. Never take a child across a road when it is unsafe, i.e. when traffic lights are on amber, when you can see a car approaching but may think it is going slowly, or from the side of parked vehicles which may restrict a driver seeing you. If children are exposed to consistently good examples of how to behave when crossing the road they will find it easier when they are older and have to learn to cross roads by themselves.

When taking children on an outing it is important that this is properly organized, whether it is a day out from the nursery or a small group of children going to the local shop to buy cooking ingredients

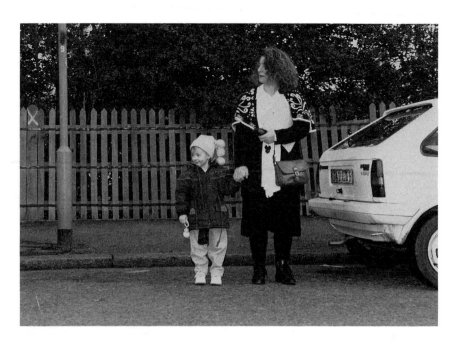

or pet food. Always check the nursery policy on taking children off the premises before embarking on any outing. In many establishments it requires parental permission in order to take a child off the premises. In some cases, members of staff may also need the permission of their line manager in order to take children off the premises.

There must always be a sufficient number of adults to cope with the number of children going out, and the minimum ratio for this can be obtained from the local authority registration officer if it is written down as part of the nursery or playgroup policy. In many instances parents may agree to accompanying a group on an outing and this will increase the number of adults available to help. All outings should be planned in advance and parents/guardians given full details in a letter about what is happening, when it is going to happen, length of the visit/outing and an invitation for them to join the outing. The bottom section of the letter can be a returnable permission slip which parents/guardians need to sign.

Any outing with children needs to be well planned. It is always a good idea to visit the place you are going to in advance so that you can be sure of the facilities that are available and the areas which may be a danger to children, and can identify suitable places that can be used as meeting points if the party becomes separated.

It is very important that the organizer of the outing has a full list of all the children that are going on the outing. It is also a good idea to make name badges for all the children. Trying to cope with a very large group can be difficult; it is much easier to split the children into smaller groups and give the adults a specific group to be responsible for. The person in charge of the outing needs to be sure that all necessary equipment is ready before the day of the outing and to decide who will be responsible for this on the day. Items such as tissues, spare clothing, sports equipment, small first aid kit etc. are the type of things that may be needed.

Transportation may be booked in advance, e.g. minibus, coach or public transport. If private cars are being used the children should travel in the back seats and be secured by seat belts or special child seats. Car doors should have childproof looks. If public transport is to be used the organizer should undertake a 'dummy run' in advance in order to identify any potential hazards or parts of the journey which may be difficult. It is essential that the person leading the party knows exactly where they are going and how they are going to get there. It is sensible to write this down for all the accompanying staff and helpers so that in the event of the party being separated, all those involved will know how to reach the final destination.

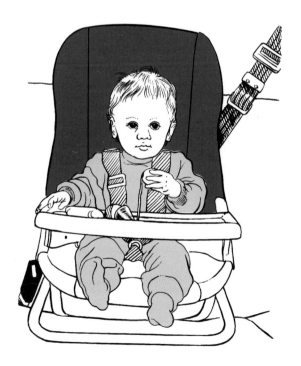

Scenario 3.2

You have been asked to move into a friend's house for 3 weeks in order to dog-sit whilst she is on holiday. You will be taking your 18-month-old daughter with you. Before moving into the house you make a visit to check that it is safe for your daughter. What will you be looking for? Describe what you will need to do in order to make this a safe environment for your daughter.

EMERGENCY SITUATIONS

Every carer hopes that they will never be in the situation to have to face an emergency but it is their duty as a responsible person to ensure that they would know what to do should such a situation arise. The most important thing in an emergency is to stay calm and not panic. The worker's first duty is to the children in their care, not their own safety, although it must be remembered that they will be no use to the children if they put their own safety in jeopardy by trying to take unnecessary heroic action.

It is essential that the person looking after the child has up-to-date and accurate records of how to contact the child's parents. This applies to all child care workers, even nannies, who must have the workplace contact number for at least one of the parents.

All child care establishments should have regular fire drills, and all staff should know how to evacuate the children quickly and safely in the event of an emergency. The action to take in the event of a fire should be clearly displayed in the nursery or playgroup, and all staff should make themselves familiar with these instructions. Staff should also know the position of fire extinguishers and know where special extinguishers are located e.g. those for electrical fires. Exits which are designated as fire exits should be clearly marked and must never be blocked by equipment or furniture.

All child care establishments and childminders should maintain an accident book. Any injuries or accidents, however minor, to staff or children are recorded in this book. In each establishment there will be a specific person who is responsible for keeping the accident book. Records of accidents should contain the date and time that the accident happened, the name of the child/staff member who had the accident, which staff member was present at the time of the accident, what type of accident occurred, what the injuries were and who gave first aid. It is useful for all child care workers to have taken a first aid course. These may be organized by the St. John's Ambulance Service or the British Red Cross, or a local college may run its own short course. All establishments should have a named first-aider who has gained a diploma in dealing with accidents at work. Most of the first aid awarding bodies require their diplomas to be updated every 3–5 years.

Whenever a child has an accident it is important to comfort and reassure them, however minor the injury may seem. All accidents must be reported to parents. In the event of a serious accident occurring the child care worker should inform whoever is in charge of the nursery or playgroup and this responsible person will then call a doctor or ambulance and inform the parents. Where the child care worker is in sole charge then they will be responsible for deciding on the seriousness of the injury, calling a doctor or ambulance and informing the parents.

Scenario 3.3

Julia is a childminder caring for Sean aged 3 years and Sophie aged 1 year. Julia has teenage sons, Rory and Malcolm. The children are with Rory and Malcolm in the sitting room watching TV whilst Julia is in the kitchen preparing tea. Rory puts his cup of hot tea on the coffee table and he does not notice Sophie crawling nearby. Before Rory realizes it, Sophie has pulled the cup of hot tea over herself and is screaming. What action must Julia and Rory take to deal with this emergency?

DEALING WITH STRANGERS

As children get older (3–8 years) they will need to be alerted to other dangers which are outside the home. Unfortunately we do not live in a safe society; not all adults that children encounter will have the child's safety at heart. It is important that children are made aware of these dangers without alarming the children or making them frightened when they meet any new adult. Leach (1989) points out that it is not always useful to tell children not to talk to strangers when we are not able to identify for them who these strangers are. It is very difficult to describe to a child exactly who counts as a friend and who counts as a stranger. Leach advocates that it is better to tell a child never to go anywhere with anybody without telling their parent or carer where they are going. This takes the decision out of the child's hands and also ensures that the child feels secure in knowing where their parent or carer is. This advice seems very sensible and can be started at an early age. As children get older they do want more freedom, but this must be balanced with ensuring that children are kept safe. Unfortunately, it is frequently the case that those people who do abuse children are not strangers to the child or the family. Many schools and playgroups use organizations such as Kidscape (address at the back of the book) to teach children how to keep themselves safe. Kidscape will send a specially trained worker to carry out training sessions with the children. All child care establishments should have a policy regarding the collection of children. Children should not be allowed to leave the premises with a person who is unauthorized to collect them. If the parent has made arrangements for a different person to collect the child then the carer must be told in advance.

KEEPING CHILDREN SAFE FROM ABUSE

Child abuse has always been present in our society but it has not always been defined or recognized as damaging to the child. The first physical child abuse case was brought before a USA court in 1857 (Allen and Morton, 1961) and had to be brought under laws pertaining to the cruelty of animals as there were no laws relating to the abuse of children. This famous case led to the founding of the National Society for the Prevention of Cruelty to Children (NSPCC) and the first laws to protect children from physical abuse were passed in 1889.

In 1968 Professor Kempe, an American paediatrician, put forward the idea of the 'battered child syndrome' and he stated that there were four factors present in child abuse cases:

1. The parents must have a background of emotional or physical deprivation and perhaps abuse as well
2. A child must be seen as unlovable or disappointing
3. There must be a crisis
4. There are no effective sources of aid at the moment of crisis

Research since the 1960s has shown that child abuse is a far more complex matter than the four factors offered by Kempe.

As society has come to learn more about child abuse it has become easier for those working with children to recognize the signs and obtain help for the family. Statistics are now kept, and with these and the high profile which the media has given to serious abuse cases, it would appear to be a prevalent problem within our society. It is difficult to prove that child abuse was common in the past as there are no statistics or records; however, some forms of child abuse are well documented in fictional works by people such as Dickens and in the work that Shaftesbury and Barnardo were doing.

There are a number of definitions of the different types of child abuse and each local authority will have these listed in their child protection documentation. The Open University uses the NSPCC definitions with some enhancements to include examples, as follows:

Neglect   Where parents (or whoever else is caring for the child) fail to meet the basic essential needs of children, like adequate food, clothes, warmth and medical care. Leaving young children alone and unsupervised is another example of neglect; refusing or failing to give adequate love and affection is a case of emotional neglect.

Physical Abuse   Where a parent (or somebody else caring for the child) physically hurts, injures or kills a child. This can involve hitting, shaking, squeezing, burning and biting. It also involves giving a child poisonous substances, inappropriate drugs and alcohol and attempted suffocation and drowning. It includes the excessive use of force when carrying out tasks like feeding or nappy changing.

Sexual Abuse   When adults seek sexual gratification by using children (boys or girls). This may be by having sexual intercourse or anal intercourse (buggery), engaging with the child in fondling, masturbation or oral sex; and includes encouraging children to watch sexually explicit behaviour or pornographic material, including videos.

Emotional Abuse   Where children are harmed by constant lack of love and affection, or threats, verbal attacks, taunting or shouting.

(Open University, 1989)

In addition to the above definition the Department of Health defines one more category:

Grave Concern   This category should not be used lightly and should be needed only in exceptional circumstances for children whose situations do not currently fit the above categories. This may be where there is an explicit and serious concern that the child is not developing as would be expected (and all medical causes have been eliminated) or there is sudden, unexplained change in that child's normal behaviour pattern. If the cause of the child's condition is later established as fitting one of the above categories, a case conference should amend the cause of registration.

(Department of Health, 1991)

Indicators of Physical Abuse

- Unexplained bruising in places where an injury cannot easily be sustained or explained
- Facial bruising
- Hand or finger marks or pressure bruising
- Bite marks
- Burns (particularly cigarette burns), scalds

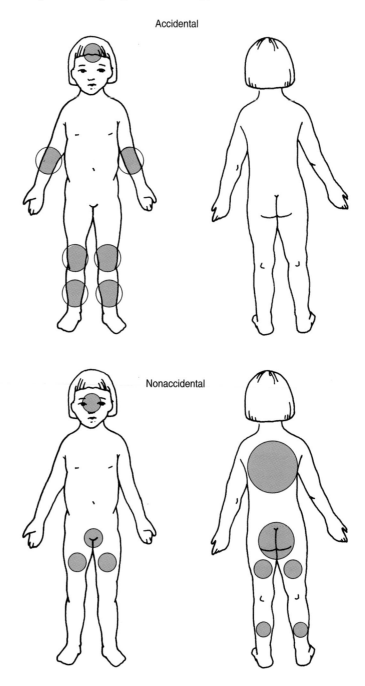

Accidental

Nonaccidental

Sites of injuries to children: accidental and non-accidental.

- Unexplained fractures
- Lacerations or abrasions

Behavioural Indicators of Physical Abuse

- Shying away from physical contact
- Withdrawn or aggressive behaviour
- Sudden changes in behaviour, e.g. from extrovert to introvert

Indicators of Sexual Abuse

- Bruises or scratches inconsistent with accidental injury
- Difficulty in walking or sitting
- Pain or itching in the genital area
- Torn, stained or bloody underclothes
- Bedwetting, sleep disturbances
- Loss of appetite

Behavioural Indicators of Sexual Abuse

- Hints of sexual activity through words, play, drawings etc.
- Sexually precocious, uses seductive behaviour towards adults
- Uses sexually explicit language
- Excessive pre-occupation with sexual matters
- Informed knowledge of adult sexual behaviour
- Poor self-esteem
- Withdrawn or isolated from other children

ROLE OF THE CARER IN CHILD PROTECTION

Child care workers are not child protection experts or child psychologists and should not attempt to play these roles. Child care workers are able to help children by listening to them, observing them and reporting their findings to the appropriate person so that the child can get the help that it needs. Children that have suffered abuse are vulnerable and this must be remembered when carers deal with these children.

The child care worker may or may not know which children in their care are designated as 'at risk' from abuse. If a child care worker does have information about a child's 'at risk' status then they must maintain strict confidentiality on this matter at all times. It is not always easy to spot signs of child abuse and for the carer the most indicative sign that something is wrong with a child is a change in the child's behaviour. However, the carer must beware of jumping to conclusions as child abuse is not the only reason for a change in a child's behaviour. A major role of the child care worker is to observe the children in their care and report anything which may give the carer cause for concern. It is a good idea to observe a child on a number of occasions during the day and write down these observations. At the end of the day these observations can be discussed with the carer's immediate superior or co-worker.

If a carer finds bruising or other physical signs on a child during the routine process of changing a child's clothes then they must report this immediately to their superior. All carers should be aware of the local authority child protection policy. If a child discloses information to their carer this must be treated with sensitivity. At no time should the worker tell the child that they do not believe them. As the Department of Health document *Working Together* (1991) states:

> A child's statement about an allegation of abuse, whether in confirmation or denial, should always be taken seriously. A child's testimony should not be regarded as inherently less reliable than that of an adult. However, professionals need to be aware that a false allegation may be a sign of a disturbed family environment and an indication that the child may need help.

The carer should tell the child that they believe them and that they are glad that they have told them. The carer should also express sympathy and sadness that it has happened to the child. The child may feel that it is their fault and will therefore need reassurance. Carers are there to listen to the child and report what they have heard; they must not press the child for details or question them. The carer should also tell the child that they will do their best to protect them and help them in the future.

Assignments

1. Plan an outing for a small group of 3-year-olds. The plan should include all the preparations that need to be made in advance and on the day.

2. Describe accurately, including diagrams and room layouts, the procedures you would take when you hear the fire alarm in your workplace.

3. You are supervising outdoor play when Gemma, aged 3 years, falls down the steps on the slide. What immediate action do you take? What follow-up action may be required?

4. Describe how you would teach a small group of 4-year-olds about road safety.

5. Describe the role of the child care worker in relation to child protection.

REFERENCES AND FURTHER READING

Allen, Anne and Morton, Arthur (1961). *This is Your Child: the story of the National Society for Prevention of Cruelty to Children*. Routledge & Kegan Paul, London.

Bray, Madge (1991). *Poppies on the Rubbish Heap: sexual abuse: the child's voice*. Canongate, Edinburgh.

Butler-Sloss, Elizabeth (1987). *Report of the Inquiry into Child Abuse in Cleveland*. HMSO, London.

Campbell, Beatrix (1988). *Unofficial Secrets, Child Sexual Abuse: the Cleveland case*. Virago, London.

Child Accident Prevention Trust (1994). *Accident Prevention in Day Care and Play Settings: a practical guide*. Child Accident Prevention Trust, London.

Children's Legal Centre (1988). *Child Abuse Procedures: the children's viewpoint*. Children's Legal Centre, London.

Department of Health (1991). *Working Together*. HMSO, London.

Elliott, Michelle (1991). *Feeling Happy, Feeling Safe: a safety guide for young children*. Hodder and Stoughton, London.

Griffin, Sue (1994) *Keeping and Writing Records: a step-by-step guide for early years workers*. VOLCUF Starting Points No 17. VOLCUF, London.

Kempe, Ruth and Kempe, Henry (1978) *Child Abuse*. Fontana, London.

Leach, Penelope (1989). *Baby and Child*. Penguin, London.

Leach, Penelope (1992). *Young Children Under Stress*. VOLCUF Starting Points No 13. VOLCUF, London.

O'Hagan, Maureen and Smith, Maureen (1993). *Special Issues in Child Care*. Baillière Tindall, London.

Open University (1989). *Unit P554: Child Abuse and Neglect: Course Materials*.

VOLCUF (1990) *Child Abuse: a guide for under fives workers*. VOLCUF, London.

Wolfe, Linda (1993) *Safe and Sound: A complete guide to first aid and emergency treatment for children and young adults*. Hodder and Stoughton, London.

Chapter 4

Diet and Nutrition

This chapter covers underpinning knowledge for parts of the following unit for the National Vocational Qualifications (NVQs) in Child Care and Education: C2
Also linked to CACHE awards modules: Diploma Modules K; Certificate Module: 5

INTRODUCTION

It is essential for children to have a well balanced diet if they are to thrive and develop physically and intellectually. The food that we eat supplies the essential nutrients needed for energy and growth. In recent years there has been emphasis placed upon the healthy diet, with high profile media attention being given to healthy eating. Many more people are turning to vegetarianism for environmental or economic reasons and it is not uncommon to find children coming into nursery or school who are vegetarians for non-religious reasons. Parents are now more aware about the food that they give to their children and the harmful effects of so-called 'junk' foods. However, we live in a 'fast food' society where it is often cheaper and easier to buy a ready prepared meal than purchase the individual ingredients to make the same meal at home. In our society good food is expensive and a child's diet is likely to reflect the income of the family. Poor families may be forced to opt for the less nutritious but more filling foods such as bread, cakes, biscuits because these are cheaper. Purchasing the ingredients to make the food is just one aspect of producing the meal as it will still need to be cooked, and the prices of gas and electricity are high. Research carried out by Dobson *et al.* (1994) interviewed families living on low incomes and the process by which these families decided what foods to eat. The following are some of the findings from this research:

◆ Families changed their food-buying habits in order to economize. The cost of food took precedence over taste, cultural acceptability and healthy eating
◆ Mothers had to ration their supplies, decide where to shop, and not give in to temptation. Shopping became unenjoyable and they derived little pleasure from eating

◆ Families tended to shop little and often at local discount super-markets

◆ Parents were concerned that their children should not be seen as different from their peer group and in order to maintain this gave them crisps or chocolate to take to school

Whilst 'junk' foods such as crisps, chips, soft drinks, sweets and biscuits are harmful to children's teeth and may lead to overweight, there have been good cases made by nutritionists that pizzas, hamburgers, fish fingers etc. are not harmful to children.

Most child care establishments now take a great deal of care over the menus which they devise for the children in order to ensure that, whilst offering a well balanced diet, they also take into account children's preferences, the popularity of ethnic foods and the provision of vegetarian meals which appeal to children's tastes.

Britain is a pluralistic society and this is now reflected in the diet of many families. Dishes such as pizzas, curries, Chinese spare ribs, stir-fry vegetables, spaghetti, lasagne etc. are popular and feature very largely in the ready meals which are available in the frozen food sections of stores. Children enjoy these meals, which offer healthy alternatives to crisps, burgers, fish fingers and chips.

NUTRITIONAL INFORMATION

Calories

All foods contain calories, although different types of food will have different calorific values (see Table 4.1). A calorie represents the amount of energy that is produced when the body burns up the food. A calorie is a standard unit for measuring heat. It is the amount of heat energy required to raise the temperature of 1 g of water by 1°C. A kilocalorie is equal to the amount of heat energy required to raise the temperature of 1 kg of water by 1°C. Any surplus calorie intake that is not converted to energy remains in the body, leading to overweight.

Table 4.1 Energy value of food

Nutrient	Energy supplied per gram
Carbohydrate	4 kcal
Protein	4 kcal
Fat	9 kcal

Insufficient calorie intake will lead to the body not having enough calories to form the energy that is needed, and when this happens the body will draw upon its reserves to supply the energy, which results in weight loss. A child aged 2 years requires about 1000–2000 calories per day (Duff, 1994).

Water

Water is essential to life in both the plant and animal world. Water is a component of every cell. In humans, water is needed to transport elements to cells, for the removal of body waste and to aid digestion. Some water is present in the food we eat but the greatest source of water for the body is drinking water, coffee, tea, milk, soft drinks etc. A lack of water leads to dehydration, a very serious condition for small babies and young children which, if untreated, can result in death.

Protein

Proteins provide the body with the essential amino-acids which are required for growth, repair of tissue and the production of antibodies, hormones and enzymes. Animal protein is the commonest source of protein in meat-eating societies. Vegetable proteins found in pulses/legumes such as lentils, peas, beans (e.g. soya, mung daal) and chick peas do not contain all the required amino-acids; they are also less digestible and need to be consumed in much larger quantities in order to obtain the same amount of amino-acids as would be supplied by animal protein. It is therefore important that careful attention is given to children on vegetarian diets to ensure that they receive an adequate intake of protein.

Other foods which are a source of protein are milk (casein), eggs, cheese and fish.

Carbohydrates

These are energy-providing foods and they are stored in the liver in the form of glycogen. If there is too much carbohydrate in the diet to be stored as glycogen the remainder becomes body fat. Foods which are sources of carbohydrates are milk (lactose) and the 'starchy' foods such as cereals, pasta, bread, cakes etc. One of the greatest sources of carbohydrates is sugar and sweet foods. Too much sugar in the diet can lead to tooth decay and overweight.

Scenario 4.1

Mary is a childminder and has just agreed to care for Ranjit aged 2½ years. Ranjit's family are members of the Hindu religion, although both his mother and father were born in the UK. What information will Mary need to obtain from Ranjit's parents about his diet and eating habits in order to ensure that he has an easy transition from home to childminder?

Fats

These have a high calorific value in small quantities so are a good source of energy. Fats are essential as carriers of the fat-soluble vitamins (A, D, E, K); however, excess fat in the diet can lead to heart disease and obesity. Health educationalists make clear distinctions between the dangers of saturated fats, which are those found in meat and dairy products, and the healthier monosaturated fats which are found in olive and rapeseed oil and polyunsaturated fats which are found in vegetable oils, fish oils, margarine etc. Duff (1994) points out that the Department of Health recommend that fat should only be 30% of the total energy foods intake and of this, 10% should be saturated fats, 12% should be monosaturated fats and 6% should be polyunsaturated fats.

Fibre

Dietary fibre is highest in the following foods: bran, wholemeal bread, the fibrous parts of vegetables and fruit, root vegetables, peas, beans and cereals which have not been refined. Fibre is required in the diet in order to give bulk to food as it is the part of food which is not digested by the body. Fibre stimulates the bowel action and prevents constipation, provided that additional fluid intake accompanies any additional fibre that may be added to the diet. However, it is pointed out by the DHSS (1988) that high fibre diets are not recommended for children under 5 years.

Vitamins

These are essential for growth and maintenance of the body. They cannot be manufactured by the body (except vitamin D) and so need to be obtained from the food that we eat. There are two types of vitamins:

◆ Fat soluble (A, D, E, K)
◆ Water soluble (B, C)

Vitamin A

Excess is stored in the liver.

◆ *Essential for:* good vision, healthy skin, formation of tooth enamel, resistance to infection
◆ *Sources:* liver, butter, whole milk, egg yolks, green vegetables, carrots, ripe tomatoes, fish liver oils, fortified margarine, apricots
◆ *Symptoms of deficiency:* night glare and night blindness, rough scaly skin, poor tooth formation, eye inflammations

Vitamin B complex

There are a number of vitamins in the vitamin B group:

◆ Vitamin B_1 (thiamine)
◆ Vitamin B_2 (riboflavin)

- Vitamin B_3 (nicotinic acid)
- Vitamin B_6 (pyridoxine)
- Vitamin B_{12} (cyanocobalamin)
- Folic acid

Each of the above has a different chemical structure but acts in a similar way in the body. Vitamin B is used by the body to utilize proteins, carbohydrates and fats. Vitamin B is water soluble and is not stored in the body, any excess being excreted in the urine. Only the two most commonly known B vitamins (B_1 and B_2) will be looked at in any detail.

Vitamin B_1 (thiamine)

- *Essential for:* functioning of nervous tissue, production of enzyme that uses carbohydrates
- *Sources:* wholegrain cereals, nuts, peanut butter, eggs, wholemeal bread, milk and dairy foods, wheatgerm/brewer's yeast
- *Symptoms of deficiency:* fatigue, constipation, depression, irritability.

Vitamin B_2 (riboflavin)

- *Essential for:* same as for B_1
- *Sources:* milk, dairy foods, liver, meat, pulses/legumes, eggs, whole grain cereals, green leafy vegetables, wheatgerm/brewer's yeast
- *Symptoms of deficiency:* burning/itching eyes, blurred/dimmed vision, eyes sensitive to the light, inflammation of the lips and tongue, greasy/scaly skin

Vitamin C

It is water soluble and can be destroyed by heat.

- *Essential for:* formation of teeth, bones and blood vessels, growth, healthy connective tissue
- *Sources:* fresh fruit (especially citrus fruits and blackcurrants), fruit juices, tomatoes, vegetables (especially raw green) – e.g. cabbage, broccoli, peppers, potatoes
- *Symptoms of deficiency:* scurvy (sore mouth, stiff aching joints, lassitude), impaired wound healing, bleeding gums

Vitamin D

It is fat soluble and is stored in the liver.

- *Essential for:* absorption of calcium and phosphorus which are needed for the formation of bones and teeth
- *Sources:* animal only – fatty fish such as halibut or cod, fish liver oils, egg yolk; it is added to margarine. Vitamin D can also be obtained from the action of sunlight on a substance in the skin called ergosterol

◆ *Symptoms of deficiency:* rickets/osteomalacia, poor tooth development, bowed legs, soft bones

Vitamin E

The functions of this vitamin are not fully understood. It is fat soluble.

◆ *Sources:* vegetable oils, green leafy vegetables, egg yolk, milk fat, nuts, wheatgerm
◆ *Symptoms of deficiency:* as the functions of vitamin E are unknown it is not possible to diagnose a deficiency

Vitamin K

It is fat soluble and can only be absorbed if bile salts are present.

◆ *Essential for:* the clotting process of the blood
◆ *Sources:* green leafy vegetables, cauliflower, liver, soya bean oil
◆ *Symptoms of deficiency:* haemorrhagic disease of the newborn, prolonged blood clotting time

Scenario 4.2

David is a nursery officer in the toddler room of an inner city community nursery. David has recently noticed that Phillip aged 2 years has been refusing to eat his lunch. What should David do to find out the cause of Phillip's lack of appetite and how can he help Phillip regain an interest in food?

Minerals

These are elements, other than carbon, hydrogen and oxygen, which are essential for all bodily functions and growth and development. There are seven essential minerals: calcium, iodine, iron, phosphorus, potassium, sodium and zinc. The most likely of these to be lacking in the diet are calcium, iron, iodine and possibly zinc.

Calcium

◆ *Essential for:* healthy bones and teeth in association with vitamin D and phosphorus), also the clotting process of blood
◆ *Sources:* milk, cheese, mustard, broccoli, cauliflower, cabbage, molasses, clams, oysters
◆ *Symptoms of deficiency:* rickets/osteomalacia, porous bones, bowed legs, stunted growth, tetany

Iodine

◆ *Essential for:* production of thyroxine in the thyroid gland
◆ *Sources:* iodized salt, seaweeds, sea foods, vegetables grown in regions close to the sea

    ◆ *Symptoms of deficiency:* cnlargcd thyroid gland (goitrc), low mcta-bolic rate, stunted growth, retarded mental growth

Iron

Absorption of iron is aided by vitamin C. Babies are born with a store of iron in their liver.

    ◆ *Essential for:* formation of haemoglobin in the blood
    ◆ *Sources:* red meat, liver, green vegetables, prunes, raisins, egg yolk, potatoes, wholegrain cereals, curry powder, sardines, haddock, cocoa
    ◆ *Symptoms of deficiency:* nutritional anaemia, pallor, weight loss, fatigue, weakness, retarded growth

Phosphorus

Works in conjunction with Vitamin D and calcium.

    ◆ *Essential for:* maintenance of body fluids, cell structure, formation of bones and teeth
    ◆ *Sources:* milk, cheese, egg yolk, fish, nuts, pulses/legumes, whole-grain cereals
    ◆ *Symptoms of deficiency:* rickets/osteomalacia, porous bones, bowed legs, stunted growth

Potassium

Works with sodium and can be lost during bouts of severe diarrhoea or if diuretics are used.

    ◆ *Essential for:* maintenance of body fluids
    ◆ *Sources:* wholegrain cereals, meat, potatoes, pulses/legumes, liver, fish, yeast extract, milk chocolate
    ◆ *Symptoms of deficiency:* apathy, muscular weakness, cardiac arrest, tachycardia (fast pulse rate)

Sodium

Babies cannot tolerate a high sodium intake due to the immaturity of their kidneys, therefore extra salt should never be added to their diet.

    ◆ *Essential for:* maintenance of cellular fluid, part of plasma, sweat and tears
    ◆ *Sources:* table salt, baking powder, milk, cheese, meat, egg white
    ◆ *Symptoms of deficiency:* dehydration, muscle cramps, weakness, headache, nausea
    ◆ *Symptoms of excess:* retention of water, changes in blood pressure, kidney damage

Zinc

    ◆ *Essential for:* cell growth, healing of wounds; also controls activity of 100 enzymes and is involved in the functioning of insulin

◆ *Sources:* lean meat, wholewheat bread, wholegrain cereals, pulses/legumes, seafood
◆ *Symptoms of deficiency:* poor growth, delayed sexual maturation, impairment of taste, loss of appetite, hair loss, inflammation of skin, mouth and tongue; a deficiency may be caused by a malabsorption disease

Additives

An additive is anything which is put into food that does not have a nutritional value, for example, preservatives, flavourings, flavour enhancers, colourings, thickeners, stabilizers, emulsifiers, antioxidants and sweeteners. There are over 3000 additives available to British food manufacturers. The reason that manufacturers add these to food is to make the food more attractive to the purchaser. Polunin (1984) states that additives can be put into the following groups:

1. Built-in additives such as the addition of artificial sweeteners in low calorie drinks
2. Convenience additives which make life easier for the producer as they increase the shelf-life of the product. Examples of these are the preservatives added to meat pies, and anti-mould additives in bread
3. Cosmetic additives which help the product to be more attractive to the purchaser in appearance, taste, flavour, consistency etc. A large proportion of additives in this group are colourings, flavourings, flavour enhancers etc.

In the UK, additives to food are regulated by the Ministry of Agriculture, Fisheries and Food (MAFF) and have to comply with the Food and Drugs Act and other regulations. In line with the rest of the European Union (EU) all food packages must show the name and EU number of the additives. Thus if you were reading the ingredients on a packet you may also see 'Tartrazine E102' (a food colouring), 'Sulphur dioxide E220' (a very common preservative). In recent years there have been a number of claims by researchers that there is an association between additives in food and hyperactivity in children. This idea was first put forward by Feingold in the USA, who suggested that children with over activity, short attention spans and impulsive behaviour might improve if they were given a diet which did not contain artificial colourings. Although scientists have yet to prove a causal relationship between food additives and hyperactivity, research carried out at Great Ormond Street Hospital does suggest that food additives such as tartrazine (E102), sulphur dioxide (E220), benzoic acid (E211, E212, E213) and monosodium glutamate (E621) could be associated with allergic conditions such as asthma, rashes, rhinitis and headaches.

Most parents and child care workers are aware of the possible dangers of additives and deliberately buy food and drinks for their children that do not contain numbers such as E102, E220, E211, E212, E213 and E621.

MEALTIMES

Mealtimes are part of the nursery and family routine and should happen at set times every day. There should be a pre-mealtime routine whereby the toys are packed away, children visit the toilet, wash their hands and then prior to eating may have a quiet activity such as a story. Once children are old enough they should participate in helping to lay the table ready for the meal. This activity is able to give them the mathematical experiences of learning about one-to-one correspondence, counting cutlery etc.

Mealtimes should be pleasant, relaxed social occasions for the child with their family or at the nursery with their friends and carers. There should be plenty of time for the child to feed themselves and enjoy their food in an unhurried atmosphere. Seating should be comfortable and of the right height to enable the child to reach the table. Eating utensils should be of a size and form which the child can manage. Children must always be encouraged to sit down and eat, a situation that some children may not be familiar with if they come from a

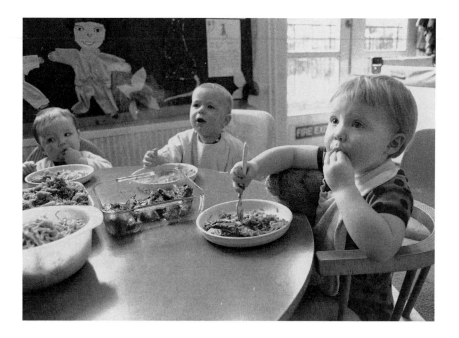

home that relies on snack meals and 'TV dinners'. A good way to encourage children to develop social skills and table manners is for the carer to sit with the children and set an example of how they should behave at mealtimes. This also enables the carer to have the children who are difficult eaters sitting near them so they can offer help and encouragement. It is useful to remember that there are different cultural aspects to mealtimes, for example, not all cultures use cutlery for eating, and using the fingers should not be frowned upon. In some cultures men and women eat separately, or children may sit together at a separate table from the adults. However, as children get used to the nursery they will want to do the same things as their friends and this will include copying the dominant eating habits.

Mealtimes are good opportunities for the child to learn new skills and develop their language, through talking about the food that is being eaten, names of vegetables, meat, fish etc. Food also introduces children to different textures and colours. New words such as smooth, lumpy, chewy, hard, soft, cooked, raw, sweet, sour etc. all help to extend a child's vocabulary and enable them to have a better understanding of their environment.

Meals should be served in an attractive manner and should contain a variety of tastes. If offering new foods to a child it is best to do this at the beginning of the meal when the child is hungry. Small portions of a new food can be introduced on a daily basis for a period of a

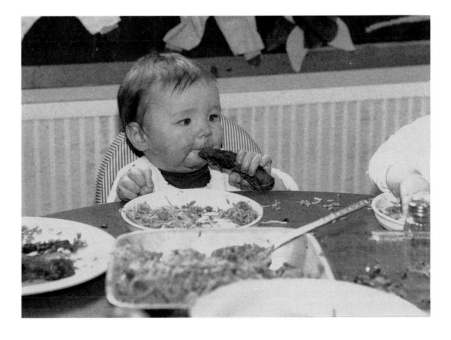

week to enable the child to gradually get used to the taste. Small children like finger foods and this is a way of introducing raw vegetables, fruit, wholemeal bread etc. into their diet. Some children only like very small portions of food and this should be respected; the carer should only give them the quantity which the child is happy with.

Children should be discouraged from eating snacks between meals as this takes away their appetite for the main meal. Many toddlers and pre-school children develop 'food fads', refusing to eat some foods or requesting the same food at every meal. There is no need to be alarmed at this as it is the child's way of gaining some independence and being able to choose what they will eat. Children should never be made to eat a food that they dislike or be force fed.

When devising menus for the nursery the children's cultural and religious backgrounds need to be taken into consideration. For example, Jews, Rastafarians and Muslims do not eat pork; Jews and Muslims can only eat meat that has been killed according to their religious laws; Hindus do not eat beef. If you are working in a multi-cultural setting it is always wise to include a vegetarian dish on the menu. However, as previously mentioned, many families are vegetarian for reasons other than religion and these parents would also expect a vegetarian meal to be available for their children.

When children start at nursery it is useful to find out from parents what their dietary requirements are, including the foods that they like

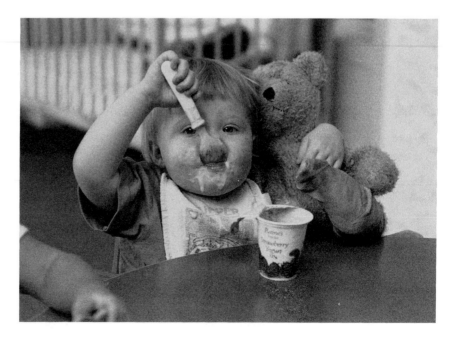

and dislike. It can also be useful to gain some knowledge from the parents as to what mealtimes are like in the home: are they used to sitting at a table, do they use a high chair etc. Some children may have food allergies, and carers need to be aware of these so they can ensure that the children are not offered the foods that cause the allergy.

There may be children with special needs in the nursery and they may need special cutlery and equipment to help them eat independently. Equipment such as cups with specially shaped feeder spouts, cutlery with chubby shaped handles, or special chairs that enable them to reach the table may be required, depending upon the special needs of the child. These children must be given every opportunity and encouragement to learn to feed themselves, even if this means that for them mealtimes are a slow process.

Scenario 4.3

Pat is a playgroup leader. Every day the children arrive at playgroup with crisps, sweets and other snacks. Pat is worried that the children are eating too much 'junk' food during the playgroup session. What strategies can Pat use for dealing with this?

FOOD HYGIENE

All people involved in the preparing of food or drinks for others who are not members of their family are required by the Food Safety Act 1990 to have a Food Handling Certificate. This is a very basic course which covers the main points attached to the hygiene of preparing and storing food. All childminders, playgroup workers and child care workers will need to gain this certificate. Environmental Health Officers from the local authority have the right to inspect all establishments where food and drinks are prepared and served.

Care should be taken in the handling of all food as bacteria can be found in cooked and uncooked foods. Most people in the UK have refrigerators for storing food; however, it is important to ensure that they are set at the correct setting so that food is stored at the right temperature. Modern fridges have an indicator inside which tells you if they are too warm. Cooked meats should be stored on the top shelves and raw meats on the bottom shelves to prevent contamination. Fresh food stored in a refrigerator should always be covered. Fridges should be defrosted regularly and thoroughly washed.

In Europe pre-packaged foods will have a number of dates printed on them, for example, a 'sell by' date, a 'best before' date and a 'use by' date. When buying food always check that it has not passed its 'sell by' date. Do not use food that has passed the 'use by' date. Food that is marked with a 'best before' date can be used after the date is passed but will probably not taste as good as the quality may have deteriorated. Some stores reduce foods on the day of the 'sell by' date; if these are purchased they should not be stored but used immediately.

Certain foods have gained a reputation for being carriers of salmonella or other types of food poisoning if they are not fully cooked, eggs and chicken being the main culprits. Raw eggs should not be given to babies, young children or other vulnerable people such as the sick or elderly. All chicken should be thoroughly cooked and particular care should be taken to ensure that the meat is cooked through to the centre. All frozen foods should be thoroughly defrosted before cooking. The use of microwave ovens has become commonplace; however, it is essential to ensure that all microwave meals are cooked all the way through. Microwave ovens come in different power strengths and it is important to ensure that the cooking time used is the right length for the power of the oven. Most microwave meals have full cooking instructions on the back of the packet. Microwaving makes food very, very hot and care must be taken to ensure that it is cooled before giving the meal to children.

Personal hygiene is important when handling food. Hands should be thoroughly washed before touching food. Any cuts or other open wounds should be covered with a waterproof dressing. The kitchen where food is prepared requires a high standard of hygiene. All surfaces should be washed down regularly using a disinfectant. Chopping boards should be colour coded with separate boards for meat and vegetables. Wooden chopping boards must be thoroughly scrubbed with a brush and detergent after every use. All cutlery, crockery and cooking utensils should be washed after use in hot soapy water, rinsed and then dried thoroughly before storing. Rubbish bins should be emptied and cleaned regularly. It is important to keep the kitchen free from flies, which contaminate the food that they come to rest on. If food is prepared in advance and left on work surfaces then it should be covered to prevent contamination.

With the present day intensive farming methods many fruits and vegetables will have come into contact with fertilizers and other chemicals. It is therefore important to wash them before using. Some fruit such as apples and lemons are given a coating of wax in order for them to look more attractive; it is important that this is removed by thorough washing before they are given to children to eat.

Assignments

1. Plan a week's menus for your nursery bearing in mind that there are children who are vegetarians, Muslims and Afro-Caribbeans.

2. What is a balanced diet? Give a full explanation of what you understand by this term and what strategies as a child care worker you can use to ensure that the children in your care receive a balanced diet.

3. Scurvy was the curse of sailors in the 17th and 18th centuries. Why do you think this disease was so prevalent amongst this group of people? What components of the daily diet in present times go towards preventing scurvy?

4. By law all pre-packaged foods must have a breakdown of their components printed on the packet. What type of components are you likely to find that may be harmful to children if eaten regularly over a long period of time? State why you have chosen a particular component and the reasons for it being harmful.

5. Devise a project for a group of 4-year-olds which will make them more aware of the meaning of healthy eating.

6. Describe how a nursery cookery session could help children have a greater understanding of their diet.

REFERENCES AND FURTHER READING

Burgess, Lynne (1995). *Cookery Activities*. Bright Ideas for Early Years Series. Scholastic, London.

DHSS (1988). *Present Day Practice in Infant Feeding*. Report on Health and Social Subjects No. 32. London, HMSO.

Dobson, Barbara, Beardsworth, Alan, Keil, Teresa and Walker, Robert (1994). *Eating on a Low Income,* Social Policy Research No 66. Joseph Rowntree Foundation, York.

Duff, Elizabeth (1994) On the sugar trail. *Nursery World*, 29 September, p. 26.

Duff, Elizabeth (1994). Vitamins. *Nursery World*, 6 October, p. 26.

Duff, Elizabeth (1994). Fat in children's diets. *Nursery World*, 13 October, p. 19.

Food Safety Advisory Centre (1993). *Food Safety Questions and Answers*. Food Safety Advisory Council, London.

Greenslade, Julie (1994). Go with the flow (importance of water in the diet). *Nursery World*, 14 April, p. 18.

Polunin, Miriam (1984). *The Right Way to Eat*. Dent and Sons, London.

Chapter 5

Working with Babies

This chapter covers underpinning knowledge for parts of the following units for the National Vocational Qualifications (NVQs) in Child Care and Education: C12, C13; there may also be some material appropriate for C14

This chapter is also linked to CACHE awards modules: Diploma Module: L; Certificate Modules: 1a, 1b

INTRODUCTION

Many jobs in the child care and education field do not require workers to have the knowledge and experience with the 0–1 year age group. This is reflected in the core modules of the National Standards (NVQs) which cover the age ranges 1–4 years and 4–7 years. However, many jobs do require a knowledge and understanding of the 0–1 year age group, for example, child minding, nannies, mother's helps, those working in settings that offer full day care where there is a baby room etc. During recent years there has been an increase in provision in the education sector for the 3–5 year age group and parents have taken advantage of this by opting to send their child to a nursery school or class. In turn this has led to the age range in nurseries and family centres falling. Many day care facilities will take children from as young as 6 months and this means that there is a need for training carers to work with this younger age range of children.

In order for a baby to feel secure it needs to be cared for by the same person or a small team of people, for example parents/childminder, parents/nanny or parents/nursery worker. If the carers of the baby are constantly changing this will lead to to the child feeling insecure. As John Bowlby (1953) pointed out in his studies on maternal deprivation, it is necessary for a baby to form attachments (bonding) with its carers and if this does not happen it may be detrimental to the child's development. The reasons for a baby failing to bond would be the lack of opportunity for the child to do this due to the absence of stable caring figures, or to constantly changing carers. A baby can bond to a number of significant people in its immediate family group such as mother, father, siblings, grandparents, aunts, uncles etc. and in addition may also form attachments with the childminder, nanny or carer. As long as these people are constant figures in the baby's life they will be able to offer consistency and continuity of care. In the early days, babies are able to identify their carers by the way they hold them, the sound of their voice and the smell of the person.

There is a myth in society that caring for babies is just about feeding, changing nappies and putting the baby down to sleep. How wrong this analysis is. The first year of life is a period of rapid growth and development physically, socially, intellectually and emotionally. It therefore takes a special person to care for a baby, someone who is able to understand and respond to the baby's verbal and non-verbal messages, someone who is able to stimulate the child so that it is able to make its first movements towards sitting and walking, make the first coos and babbles towards language development etc. Therefore babies need carers whose role is to give them a safe secure environment, stimulation and loving care and attention.

For a family, the arrival of a new baby should be a joyous event for all members. The pregnancy is a time for preparation and coming to terms with the fact that there will be extra responsibilities for the adults. All members of the family should be involved in the preparations and siblings can be encouraged to feel the mother's stomach as the baby grows and help in choosing clothing, furniture and other items for the new baby. We live in a society where contraception and abortion are available and it should follow that all babies are wanted babies. Sadly, this is not always the case, for reasons which may be very complex, not every baby will be wanted. Child care workers need to be aware of this as it may require them to work very hard to facilitate the bonding between a mother and her child.

Scenario 5.1

Sarah is on maternity leave with her first child, Siobhan. Sarah knows that in 6 weeks time she must return to work, therefore she is exploring all the available day care options in her locality. Sarah is worried about leaving Siobhan at such a young age for long periods of time, however, she has no alternative but to return to work. You are the Officer-in-Charge of the baby room in Sarah's local nursery. What would you tell Sarah about your provision that would reassure Sarah that she was doing the right thing by leaving Siobhan in your care?

PREGNANCY: SIGNS AND STAGES

A normal pregnancy lasts for 40 weeks, and this is calculated from the first day of the woman's last menstrual period. Missing a menstrual period does not automatically mean that a woman is pregnant, therefore a doctor should be consulted for confirmation of pregnancy. There are home pregnancy testing kits which can be purchased at the pharmacists (chemists); however, these are not 100% accurate and there is always a risk that they will show the wrong result.

A woman's pregnancy is divided into three trimesters, each lasting for 3 months. In the first 8 weeks following conception the baby is referred to as an embryo. After that period it is called a fetus.

First Trimester (0–12 weeks)

First signs of pregnancy are the absence of menstrual periods. The breasts start to swell and become tender, the nipples start to enlarge. Nausea and vomiting are common and often occur in the morning (morning sickness); this may last for 6–8 weeks.

Second Trimester (13–28 weeks)

From about 16 weeks the enlarging uterus is easily felt and the woman begins to look noticeably pregnant. Nipples enlarge and darken. Appetite increases and weight can rise rapidly. By about the 22nd week the woman would have felt the baby moving around (quickening).

Third Trimester (29–40 weeks)

Stretch marks may begin to develop on the woman's abdomen. Colostrum can be expressed from the nipples. More rest may be needed at this stage. The baby's head engages (drops into the low pelvis) around the 36th week in preparation for the birth.

ANTE-NATAL CARE

The purpose of ante-natal care is to monitor the health of the mother and baby. If anything is found to be amiss with either the mother or the baby it can be dealt with quickly. Good ante-natal care provided free to all mothers is a major way of preventing and lowering the maternal and infant death rates.

On the first visit to the ante-natal clinic the woman will be able to discuss the available options for her on-going care and the delivery of the baby. Depending upon the facilities available in the local health authority the woman may be able to choose between a home or hospital delivery, and whether her ante-natal care will be a shared responsibility between her GP, Community Midwife and hospital or will be totally the responsibility of the hospital. Nearer the time of her delivery the staff at the ante-natal clinic will discuss with the woman the birth positions which may be available, for example, crouching, birthing chairs, birthing pools, stirrup position etc. and the advantages and disadvantages of each. It will then be left for the woman to make up her mind and to inform the midwife of her preferences once she has gone into labour. Mothers are encouraged to actively involve their partners in the pregnancy and birth. If a woman is going through the pregnancy alone she will be encouraged to involve a close family member or friend who can act as a support for her during the ante-natal period and the birth.

Ante-natal clinics are also able to offer relaxation classes and general advice to the mother and her partner about what is happening throughout the different stages of the pregnancy and what can be expected at the onset of labour.

The first 12 weeks of pregnancy are, in many ways, the most critical as it is during this time that the baby's essential organs are being formed. Once a woman thinks that she is pregnant (although not necessarily confirmed by a doctor), it is important that she carefully considers changing any parts of her lifestyle which could be harmful to the baby. The following are examples of the things which an expectant mother may have to consider changing during pregnancy.

Smoking

It is now a well established scientific fact that smoking retards the growth of the fetus by cutting down the oxygen supply to the baby. Mothers who smoke when they are pregnant are more likely to have a low birth weight baby or a baby described as small for dates. These babies are very vulnerable and may need special care after birth. Women who smoke should do everything possible to give up smoking during the pregnancy. This will take a lot of willpower and the woman will need support from her family and friends. Many GP group practices have special clinics to help people give up smoking and she may find it easiest to attend one of these.

Alcohol

Excessive regular intake of alcoholic drinks by a woman who is pregnant can lead to a low birth weight baby. Alcohol in the bloodstream of the mother is able to cross the placenta and have an effect upon the development of the baby. Women who are alcoholics and who continue to drink during their pregnancy are at risk of having a baby which has fetal alcohol syndrome; this not only gives the child distinctive features but also leads to mental retardation.

Diet

Pregnant women need a well balanced diet. The old wives' saying of 'eating for two' is not true as it is the quality of the food and type of food consumed which is important, not the quantity. During the pregnancy the woman should gain about 12.7 kg and 70% of this weight increase should occur during the last 20 weeks of the pregnancy. There should be a daily intake of each of the following: protein, fruit, vegetables, fats, dairy products, cereals and whole grains. There should also be an adequate fluid intake as this prevents constipation. If the woman has a well balanced diet she should not need any vitamin or mineral supplements except perhaps iron, and folic acid of which 400 mcg should be taken daily throughout the first trimester at least. Vegetarians that do not eat fish, eggs or cheese (vegans) need to take special care with their diet to ensure that their protein intake is of a higher level than they would normally need.

There are some foods which are best avoided during pregnancy as they may cause listeria or salmonella poisoning and this could be harmful to the baby. Pregnant women should avoid raw or lightly cooked eggs, undercooked chicken, rare or lightly cooked meat, soft cheeses (such as Brie, Camembert) or mould ripened cheeses (such as Stilton, Roquefort, blue Brie).

Exercise

A normal amount of exercise is good for the health of the woman and the baby. However, it is not the time to take up jogging or cycling! Swimming, walking or simple exercises done on a regular basis will help the woman to keep fit. Exercise also helps to prevent constipation. The ante-natal clinic will offer exercise classes but these are specifically related the labour and post-labour period.

Dental care

Dental treatment is free during pregnancy and up until the baby is 1 year old. The mother's dental health depends a great deal upon her diet and foods rich in protein, calcium, phosphorus and vitamins A, C and D are important (the future teeth of the baby are laid down during the early months of pregnancy and therefore the mother's diet during this time will also affect the quality of the child's teeth). Teeth that are decaying can cause infections and these in turn might be harmful to the baby; it is therefore important that pregnant women take advantage of the free dental treatment which is offered to them.

Drugs

It is important that once a woman thinks that she may be pregnant she should stop taking any drugs, even those that have been prescribed for her. Women on a permanent drug regime, such as diabetics, asthmatics or epileptics, should consult their GP immediately. Doctors have a great deal of experience in monitoring women who are on permanent drug regimes. Drugs, like alcohol, are able to cross the placenta and could have serious harmful effects upon the baby.

Drug addicts who become pregnant must also contact their

doctors who will be able to offer them advice and counselling to help them give up the drugs and may also be able to offer less potent substitutes for the hard drugs that the woman may be addicted to. It is not uncommon for babies that are born to drug addicts to suffer withdrawal symptoms following the birth.

X-rays

X-rays can be harmful to the developing foetus. In the majority of hospitals the radiographer, before taking an X-ray, will always check with female patients as to whether they think they could be pregnant. If a woman suspects that she might be pregnant and is sent for an X-ray she should always tell the radiographer.

Rubella (German Measles)

For a woman to contract rubella in the first trimester (3 months) of pregnancy can cause damage to the development of the foetus. Such damage may result in the baby being born deaf, blind or mentally or physically handicapped. Since 1970 there has been a vaccination programme in secondary schools in the UK whereby teenage girls are given rubella vaccine. This has led to a dramatic fall in the numbers of children being born with rubella-associated handicaps. However, it should be noted that any woman who did not have their secondary school education in the UK may not have had the benefit of this vaccine and should therefore be warned of the dangers of contracting rubella during pregnancy. For this reason, parents of children who contract rubella should make sure that all the adult females that the child has had contact with are made aware that the child has rubella.

ANTE-NATAL SCREENING

The Health of the Mother

On the first visit to the ante-natal clinic there will be a number of screening tests that will be carried out on the mother. At this stage of the pregnancy these will be done in order to ascertain the state of health of the mother.

Blood screening

On the first ante-natal visit a sample of the mother's blood will be taken. This will be screened for the following:

◆ Blood group
◆ Rhesus factor
◆ Syphilis
◆ Viral hepatitis
◆ Rubella immunity
◆ Sickle cell disease
◆ Thalassaemia

◆ Haemoglobin level
◆ AIDS/HIV (for those women who think they may have been at risk)

On the initial visit and subsequent visits the mother will also undergo urine screening.

Urine screening

A urine sample will be taken from the mother every time that she visits the ante-natal clinic. This sample will be tested for:

◆ Sugar
◆ Protein
◆ Ketones

Blood pressure and weight will also be taken at each visit. If the woman registers a low haemoglobin count in the first blood test, further tests may be taken at subsequent ante-natal visits throughout the pregnancy.

Ultrasound Screening

Most pregnant women will be automatically given an ultrasound scan around 16–18 weeks of the pregnancy. This test is done by transmitting high frequency sounds, which cannot be heard, to the womb (it is the same method that is used to detect submarines). As the sounds bounce back they can be captured on a screen to form a picture of the baby in the womb. This test is quite harmless to the mother and baby and does not cause discomfort or distress. Ultrasound scanning can confirm the number of weeks of the pregnancy, whether there is more than one baby, that the baby is lying in the womb and not outside it, i.e. in a Fallopian tube, that the baby is developing normally and the position that the baby is lying in. The ultrasound scan can also determine the sex of the baby and this information can be given to the parents/family if they want to know. The sex of the baby can be important when there are inherited sex-linked conditions such as haemophilia or Duchenne's muscular dystrophy. Many hospitals are able to provide a photograph of the ultrasound scan picture so the family have a first picture of the baby.

Other Screening Tests

There are other screening tests which a pregnant woman may undergo at later dates during the pregnancy; these tests may be offered to all women or just to those who may be at risk. A woman has a choice as to whether she wishes to have these tests carried out. If the tests prove to be positive the woman then has the choice of continuing with the pregnancy or having it terminated (an abortion). If a woman has particular convictions about not wishing to have an abortion (these convictions may or may not be linked with religious beliefs) then she may not wish to have these tests carried out.

Spina bifida

This test may be offered as routine or to a woman who is in a high risk category, i.e. there is a history of spina bifida in the family or she already has a child with spina bifida. This test is carried out in the 16th week of the pregnancy. A blood sample is taken and tested for the level of alpha-fetoprotein (AFP) which may indicate that the child possibly has spina bifida. Low levels of AFP can also indicate that the child may have Down's syndrome.

Down's syndrome

The AFP test may be offered to women who are in a high risk category, i.e. over the age of 35 years, already have a Down's syndrome child or there is a history of Down's syndrome in the family. As already stated, low levels of AFP may indicate that the baby has Down's syndrome.

Amniocentesis

This test is carried out between the 14–16th week of the pregnancy. Using the ultrasound picture to guide the direction, a needle is used to draw off a sample of the amniotic fluid (this is the fluid that surrounds the baby in the womb). The amniotic fluid will contain cells from the baby and these can be tested for Down's Syndrome and some other genetic disorders. There is a 0.05% risk of a spontaneous miscarriage following an amniocentesis test.

Chorion biopsy

This test is carried out between the 7–11th weeks of the pregnancy. A sample of cells is taken from the chorionic villi which are found in the embryonic membrane (chorion). The sample of cells is then tested in order to detect genetic diseases such as cystic fibrosis, Duchenne muscular dystrophy, haemophilia, thalassaemia etc. The test is offered to women from families where there is a history of these diseases.

Scenario 5.2

Sharon is your neighbours' 16-year-old daughter. Sharon is 3 months pregnant. On talking with Sharon you discover that she has not attended any of her ante-natal clinic appointments. How would you explain to Sharon about the importance of ante-natal care and how would you best convince her that she should attend these clinics?

Multiple births

With ultrasound scanning it is now possible to detect at an early stage of the pregnancy the number of children that a woman is carrying. Fraternal twins are those formed when two eggs are fertilized at the same time, whereas identical twins are when one egg splits into two. Fraternal twins are more common than identical twins. With the latest treatments for infertility becoming more easily available there has been a proportional increase in the numbers of multiple births, particularly triplets and quads.

THE BIRTH

By the time a woman goes into labour (the term used to describe the birth process, probably called this as giving birth is hard work!) she will know whether she is having the baby at home or in hospital. She would also have been instructed at the ante-natal clinic or by her midwife as to the first signs of the onset of labour such as contractions, or the breaking of the waters (amniotic fluid) and what to do when these occur. There are three stages to labour.

Stage 1

This is the stage of dilation of the cervix. It starts with regular uterine contractions which push the baby and the sac of amniotic fluid downwards and the uterus upwards. The cervix, uterus and vagina all dilate in order to provide one continuous birth canal. During this stage the amniotic sac may burst or this may not happen until later in the proceedings.

Stage 2

This stage extends until the baby is delivered. During this stage the baby is pushed through the birth canal. Every contraction brings the baby further forward. Once the baby's head is through the rest of the baby can be eased out.

Stage 3

This is the stage following the birth of the baby and during which the placenta is expelled and the uterus contracts. Following the expulsion of the placenta the uterus continues to contract and diminishes in size in order to control the bleeding. On average the whole birth process will take up to 14 hours for a first baby and 8 hours for each subsequent birth.

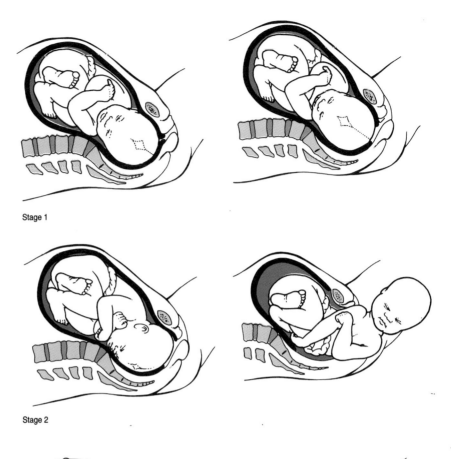

Stage 1

Stage 2

The three stages of labour.
1: onset of contractions to full
cervical dilatation (10 cm);
2: full dilatation to delivery of
infant; 3: delivery of placenta
or 'afterbirth'.

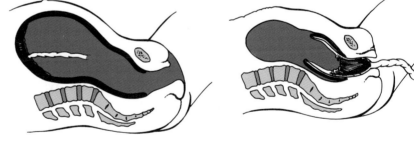

Stage 3

IMMEDIATELY FOLLOWING THE BIRTH (THE NEWBORN BABY)

The midwife will take care of the baby, cutting the umbilical cord at the beginning of the third stage of labour. The baby may have taken its first breath when the head emerges, but in some cases the midwife may have to extract mucus in the baby's mouth and throat in order to help it take this breath. The baby will be examined and given a rating known as the Apgar score (Table 5.1). This test is named after its inventor Virginia Apgar and records the heart rate, muscle tone, breathing and colour immediately following the birth.

Table 5.1 The Apgar score

Sign[a]	Score		
	0	1	2
Heart rate	Absent	Slow (below 100)	Fast (above 100)
Respiratory effect	Absent	Slow Irregular	Good Crying
Muscle tone	Limp	Some flexion of extremities	Active
Reflex irritability (stimulation of foot or oropharynx)	No response	Grimace	Cry, cough
Colour	Cyanosed Pale	Good colour Extremities blue	Very good colour

[a] The first two, heart rate and respiratory effect, are the most important.

Babies that have a low Apgar score will be carefully monitored in the first few days following the birth. Babies without difficulties usually have an Apgar score of 7–10.

All newborn babies look different and they may or may not have some of the features mentioned below.

The skin of a newborn baby is covered with a greasy film called vernix. It used to be traditional in the UK to bath the baby immediately following birth in order to wash off the vernix. However, research has shown that the vernix is best left on the baby where it is absorbed through the skin and offers the baby protection against skin infections.

The baby's face may be wrinkled and red or puffy or in some cases bruised. All these marks will disappear within the first few days following the birth.

Some babies will have a good head of dark hair which grows downwards onto the forehead. In most babies the first hair, whatever the texture and colour, will fall out and the subsequent growth of hair may bear no resemblance to the birth hair. In some religions and cultures the hair that a baby is born with is thought to be unlucky or to sap the child's future strength. In these situations the family will shave of the birth hair; this does no harm to the baby.

The body of some babies may be covered in downy hairs which are shed after the baby is about a week old.

Once the midwife has checked the baby it will be wrapped up and given to the mother to hold. At this point some midwives will encourage the mother to put the baby to the breast.

EXAMINATION OF THE NEWBORN

In the first 24 hours following the birth a doctor will usually give the baby a thorough examination.

Basic Measurements

The length of the baby and the circumference of the baby's head is measured, and the baby is then weighed. The average weight of a new-born baby is 2.5–4.4 kg (5½–9½lb), the average length is 45–55 cm (18–22 inches) and the head circumference should be about 35 cm (14 inches). A baby may lose weight following the birth but the original birthweight should be regained by the tenth day.

Head and Neck

The doctor will check the fontanelle (soft spot) on the top of the head and check for any swelling (caput) on parts of the scalp caused by pressure during the birth.

The Face

The baby's face is examined in order to check for abnormalities such as a hare lip or cleft palate, which would result in difficulties in feeding. The doctor will also check the fold of skin which holds the tongue to the floor of the mouth to ensure that it is not too short. Vision and hearing are checked by watching the child's response to light and sound.

The Heart

The heart is checked using a stethoscope. The doctor listens for abnormal heart sounds such as 'murmurs', and checks the baby's lips and nails for signs of cyanosis (blue colour), both of which could indicate that the child had a congenital heart condition.

The Genitals

The doctor inspects the genitals in order to confirm that the sex of the child has been correctly stated. Male children will also be tested to ascertain whether the testicles have descended into the scrotum.

The Umbilical Cord

The cord is checked to ensure that it is drying out normally and not becoming infected. It is not uncommon to find that some babies have a hernia around the cord area; this needs no treatment and usually disappears around the age of 5 years.

Congenital Dislocation of the Hip

The doctor is able to put both the hip joints through a range of movements to determine whether the baby has dislocated a hip during the birth process. This test does not hurt the baby. If a dislocated hip is diagnosed the baby will be referred to an orthopaedic specialist for treatment.

Hands and Feet

The hands and feet are examined for extra digits, webbing between the digits and any other deformities such as talipes (club foot).

Reflexes

A baby is born with a number of reflexes which will be tested by the doctor at the post-birth examination. These reflexes are simple responses to stimuli as follows:

- ◆ *Oral:* sucking
- ◆ *Rooting:* when the baby's cheek is touched at one side of the mouth they will turn their head to the touch
- ◆ *Eyes:* blinks in response to light
- ◆ *Grasp:* will grasp a finger that is placed in the palm of their hand
- ◆ *Moro:* if the baby is startled they fling out their arms and open their hands
- ◆ *Walking:* will attempt to walk when their feet come into contact with a horizontal surface

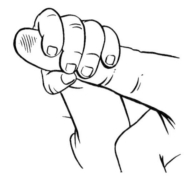 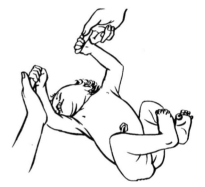

The reflex grasp and movements from lying to sitting of a newborn baby.

Premature Babies

Premature or before-term babies are those that are born before week 37 of the pregnancy. These babies will have a low birthweight, often less than 2.5 kg; be small in size with a large head and hands; the skin will be thin, shiny, smooth and will be covered in downy hair (lanugo); features may be wizened and wrinkled; veins may be visible under the skin; the abdomen will protrude; they will have a poor sucking and swallowing ability and may have a feeble whining cry.

Premature babies are at risk from respiratory distress, jaundice, poor temperature control, anaemia, low blood sugar and infection. These babies are very vulnerable and will be cared for in the Special Care Baby Unit (SCBU) usually in an incubator. An incubator provides warmth and allows easy observation of the baby; it has artificial ventilation to assist breathing. These babies will probably need to be fed artificially through a stomach tube. The baby will be kept in the incubator until they reach a weight of 2.5 kg and must be able to feed normally. Ninety percent of premature babies survive and are able to catch up with full term babies over a period of time.

Small-for-dates Babies

These are babies who have gone through the full period of pregnancy but when born have a low birthweight, under 2.3 kg (5 lb). These babies may have breathing and feeding problems and some may need to be monitored in the Special Care Baby Unit for a period of time. These babies are often born to mothers who are heavy smokers, heavy drinkers or have had poor nutrition during pregnancy.

Abilities of the Newborn

Vision

A newborn baby is able to focus on an object that is at a distance of 8–9 inches from their eyes. This distance is the amount of space between a baby feeding on the breast and the face of the mother. Professor Karmiloff-Smith of the Medical Research Council Cognitive Development Unit in London (see Reid, 1995) has found that at 4 days old an infant can recognize its mother by the shape of her face and her hair. It would appear that babies have a primitive orientation which allows them to distinguish between many different types of face. Infants gradually specialize in faces so that at the age of 2 months they prefer the whole face with all its features and at 5 months they like a moving face.

Hearing

Normally hearing babies will hear loud noises which will lead them to respond by making the Moro reflex.

Smell

A baby has a sense of smell and can recognize the smell of their mother's milk.

Touch

Many of the reflex responses of the baby are in response to touch.

Language

Recent research by Professor Annette Karmiloff-Smith (1995) has found that newborn babies can distinguish the sound of their parents'/ carer's languages from other languages which they may hear. Professor Karmiloff-Smith maintains that newborn babies are capable of distinguishing between each of the 150 speech sounds that make up all human languages, although by the age of 10 months they have lost this sensitivity.

Birthmarks

Newborn babies often have marks on their skin, the majority of which will disappear during the first few months of life.

Stork's beak marks	This term is used to describe the small pink marks which a baby may have above the bridge of the nose, on the eyelids or the nape of the neck. These usually fade over time.
Strawberry marks	These are tiny red dots which are not always obvious at first. They grow during the early months of life to become red raised lumps. They usually begin to shrink in the second year of life and may have totally disappeared by the time the child reaches school age.
Mongolian blue spot	This is the name given to a mark which is commonly found in Asian or black children but may also occur in children from other ethnic origins such as Italian, Greek, Oriental and Eskimo. It is a blue discolouration of the skin usually found on the lower back. This will fade over time. It is important that this is recognised as a birthmark and is not confused with a sign of physical abuse.
Moles (pigmented naevus)	These may be brown or blackish, flat or raised and may or may not have hairs sprouting from them. They usually appear in places where they are hidden by clothing; however, if a child has a disfiguring naevus it can be removed by plastic surgery.
Port wine stain	Of all the birthmarks found on new babies this is one of the most serious as it does not fade with time; however, it is comparatively rare. It appears as a dark red patch with sharply defined edges. It is a permanent mark and depending on where it appears may need to be dealt with in later life by the application of masking creams.
Spots and rashes	It is not uncommon for newborn babies to get spots and rashes which are usually harmless and disappear after a short time. The most common two rashes are:

◆ *Neonatal urticaria.* These are large red spots which may appear during the first week of life. They disappear after a few hours and others may appear in different places. They need no treatment and will eventually disappear altogether

◆ *Milia.* These are small white spots usually appearing on the nose. They are caused through blocked sebaceous glands. They need no treatment and will disappear of their own accord

Scenario 5.3

You are the Officer-in-Charge in the baby room of the local family centre. Shamila is an 8-month-old Asian girl in your care. Carol, the student child care worker, tells you that whilst she was changing Shamila she saw evidence of bruising on her back. What is the most likely explanation for what Carol has seen? How do you explain the situation to Carol?

FEEDING THE NEW BABY

Most mothers have a choice of breast feeding or bottle feeding their baby. However, some mothers may have physical problems which may prevent them breast feeding, e.g. needing to take drugs which will pass to the baby via the breast milk; or the baby may have physical problems which make breast feeding difficult, e.g. a cleft palate. In order for a woman to make an informed choice between breast feeding and bottle feeding the reasons for both need to be explained to her.

Reasons for breast feeding:

◆ Breast milk is a natural food, easily digestible for the baby and requires no vitamin supplements
◆ Breast milk is always at the right temperature, requires no preparation and is always available to the baby and is cheap to provide
◆ Breast milk contains antibodies which protect the baby against disease and infection

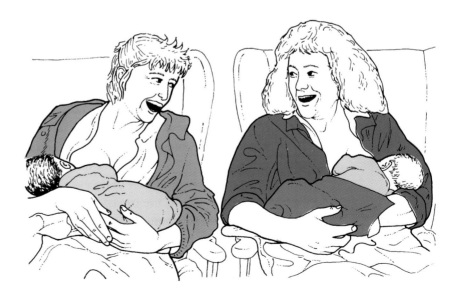

♦ Breast milk is less likely to cause the baby to have allergic reactions
♦ Breast-fed babies are not usually overweight
♦ Breast feeding helps the development of the baby's gums, teeth and jaws as the baby has to suck more vigorously in order to obtain the milk

Reasons for bottle feeding:

♦ Feeding can be shared between the mother and her partner
♦ Bottle feeding may make the mother feel more confident, particularly if they have had difficulties trying to breast feed
♦ If the woman wishes to return to work soon after the birth it may be easier to bottle-feed the baby from the beginning
♦ If it is a multiple birth situation, bottle feeding will enable others to be involved at feeding times which may make the process less stressful for the mother

Breast feeding is the recommended method of feeding a baby and most mothers are able to successfully establish breast feeding with their baby. However, there may be very valid reasons for a woman choosing to bottle-feed her baby, and the wishes of the mother should be respected.

During the first weeks of life the baby and mother together will be establishing a feeding routine. In the first instance the baby may be fed on demand and gradually this will settle down into regular periods between feeds, usually a pattern that gives the baby four to six feeds a day.

Breast Feeding

Techniques to establish breast feeding are suggested by the midwife. This is very important for first time mothers as they may lack confidence in breast feeding their baby. It is important that the mother sits/lies in a position which is comfortable for herself and the baby. The baby should be held in a comfortable way ensuring that the back of the child's neck is supported. In order for the baby to express milk from the breast it needs to be 'fixed on' to the nipple and its surrounding area. The baby holds on by suction but feeds by moving its lower jaw up and down squeezing the milk reservoirs which lie behind the nipple. The production of breast milk is on supply and demand regardless of the size of the breasts, therefore the more often the baby is put to the breast the more milk the breasts will produce. The baby should empty both breasts at each feed. If a baby is breast feeding satisfactorily it will fall asleep between feeds, gain approximately 140–225 g per week and pass soft yellow stools after the end of the first week (before this period the baby will pass what is called meconium, which is dark and sticky). Some babies take longer than others to learn to feed and the mother needs to be patient and gain advice and help from the midwife and health visitor. The La Leche League is a charitable organization which provides information, encouragement and support to women who are breast feeding. The La Leche League runs a 24 hour helpline and has local meetings (address at the back of the book).

It is important that before breast feeding a mother washes her hands. The breasts should be washed daily and if the nipples are sore a barrier cream should be applied. When the woman is breast feeding she will need a well balanced diet with plenty of liquids. She will also need to remember that whatever she takes into her body may come out in the breast milk so that strong-flavoured food such as garlic, pickled onions etc. may flavour the breast milk. Drugs and alcohol may also pass into the breast milk and great care should be taken by the breast-feeding mother over things such as laxatives, aspirin, caffeine and nicotine.

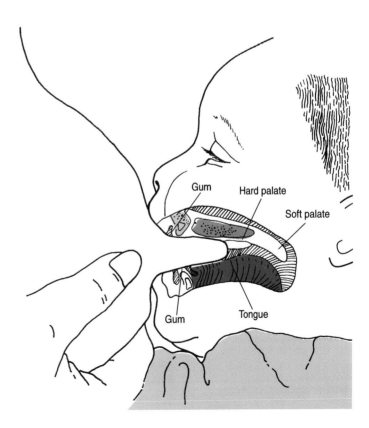

A baby breast feeding. Note that the nipple is well back in the baby's mouth.

Bottle Feeding

Babies under 6 months of age are unable to digest cow's milk. Unless the mother is expressing her own breast milk and bottle feeding her baby with this, she will need to decide which brand of dried milk formula she will use for her baby. This decision is best made in consultation with the midwife or health visitor. Most baby milk formulas are supplemented with vitamins A, B_{12}, C and D.

It is important that all the equipment used to make up bottle feeds and the bottles and teats are sterilized before use. There are a number of sterilizing agents available on the market and the instructions for using these should be followed carefully. A plastic sterilizing unit can be purchased and this will hold a number of bottles and teats. Metal implements cannot be sterilized using proprietary sterilizing agents so it is better to use plastic spoons, knives, or glass/pyrex measuring jugs. In the absence of chemical sterilizing agents the equipment should be boiled in a saucepan of water ensuring that all the equipment is fully submerged in the water and the water is kept at boiling temperature for at least 10 minutes. If this method of sterilization is used the equipment will need to be drained and allowed to cool naturally before using.

When preparing a feed using milk formula it is important to follow all the instructions which are printed on the packet. The scoop provided in the packet of milk must be used and a 'level scoop' is a scoop which has been levelled by passing a knife or other flat utensil across the top of the scoop. The scoop should be lightly filled (not packed full as this will make the feed too concentrated) and half scoop measures should not be used as they cannot be measured accurately. Sugar must not be added to the feed.

Preparing the feed

Nurseries will have a milk kitchen, which is an area separate from the main kitchen and used only for preparing bottle feeds. In the home, the person preparing the feed should use an area in the kitchen that is easy to keep scrupulously clean. When preparing a bottle feed, strict attention should be paid to cleanliness of the area where the feed is being made and the good hygiene practices of the person preparing the feed.

Before making the feed all the necessary equipment should be gathered together. You will need the milk formula, boiled water and the following previously sterilized utensils, a plastic straight edged knife, glass/pyrex jug, feeding bottle and teat. Always wash your hands before preparing the feed. Following the manufacturer's instructions on the milk formula packet, pour the required amount of boiled water into the jug, add the required amount of milk formula, stirring to ensure that there are no lumps, pour this into the feeding bottle, place the teat on the bottle and cover this with the teat protector. All the bottles needed to feed a baby for a 24 hour period can be made at the same time, storing them in the refrigerator and reheating using a microwave or a jug of hot water. It is only possible to use this method if the carer has enough bottles; feeds cannot be made in advance and kept in other containers until needed as this will lead to contamination of the feed. Place the bottle on a tray with two jugs of water, one hot and one cold. Take the tray to the room where you will be feeding the baby and place it in a safe position but within easy reach of the person who is feeding the baby. Always wash your hands before you feed a baby.

When feeding a baby it is best to sit them on your lap in a similar position to the one they would be in if they were being breast fed. **Babies should not be fed lying in cots or propped up in chairs.** Holding the baby close during feeding is part of the bonding process between the carer and child. The temperature of the milk must always be tested before giving the feed to the baby. This is done by putting a few drops of milk on the back of the adult's hand; it should not be too hot or too cold. If the feed is too hot it should be placed in the jug of cold water until it cools to the right temperature. If the feed is too cold it should be placed in the jug of hot water until it reaches the right temperature. The size of the hole in the teat should enable the baby to get a free flow of milk when it sucks hard. If the hole is too large the baby will not have to suck so hard and will miss out on strengthening its jaw muscles. When feeding the baby the bottle should be held at an angle which ensures that there is no gap between the teat and the liquid. This prevents the baby sucking in air which can result in the baby getting 'wind'. All babies take in some air during the sucking process and it is a good idea to stop the feed half way through and 'wind' the baby. This is done by holding the baby in an upright position, usually supported on the shoulder of the person feeding the baby, and gently rub the baby's back until it burps (expels the air). This also needs to be done at the end of the feed. Air trapped in the baby's stomach can be painful. After feeding the baby should have a nappy change and be put into its cot to sleep.

Following the feed all the bottle-feeding equipment needs to be thoroughly washed and placed into the sterilizing unit making sure that the sterilizing fluid gets right inside the bottles and there are no air bubbles. Bottles need to be washed using a bottle brush and should be washed in cold water first to remove milk residues and film. The same care applies to teats. The sterilizing solution needs to be changed every 24 hours. Bottle-feeding utensils are a potential source of infection and must therefore be carefully washed and sterilized before using to prepare a feed. For babies, infections such as gastroenteritis are very serious and if not treated by a doctor immediately can lead to complications and even death.

Weaning

Weaning is the term used to describe the baby's transition from bottle feeding to solid foods. (In some books it may also be used to describe the baby's transition from breast feeding to bottle feeding.) About 4–6 months of age most babies will require more food intake than they can obtain from a milk-only diet. Bottle-fed babies seem to give signs that they are dissatisfied with their feeds earlier than breast-fed babies; this may be due to the fact that the harder a breast-fed baby sucks the more milk there is available to it. Research by Dr Gill Harris from Birmingham University (see Reid, 1995) has found that babies are most receptive to a wide range of foods between 3–6 months. In some cultures, babies are weaned at a much later date; this may be due to tradition, unavailability of suitable weaning foods or economics, as breast milk is free. Research appears to show that the later a baby is weaned the less chance there is of the child having allergic reactions to certain foods. The common foods that may produce allergic reactions are cow's milk, eggs (particularly egg white), wheat, cheese, shellfish and pork. Babies should never be weaned by adding cereals to their bottle feed. The foods that are used to wean a baby will vary depending upon the culture and diet within the family. For example, the Chinese wean their babies onto a mushy rice called congee and as Leach (1988) points out, in California and Israel avocado pears are a common weaning food. What is important is that they are pure foods with no added sugar, salt or 'E' number additives. New tastes should be introduced slowly, giving the baby one new food at a time. Food needs to be mushy (puréed through a sieve) or liquidized as the baby will not have teeth to chew lumps. The food needs to be of such a consistency that the baby can suck it from the spoon. When introducing the baby to solid foods it is usual to decide on one feed, i.e. lunchtime or early evening feed, as the regular time when solids will be introduced. They can be given before or after the milk feed, although some practitioners believe that the baby may be more interested in the solid food if it is given before the milk feed. The baby can be fed whilst being held on the lap of the carer or can be sat in a high (or low) chair. A sterilized plastic teaspoon is used to give the baby the food. Make sure that the baby has a bib or other protection for their clothes as they are inclined to spit the food out or let the food dribble out of their mouths. One or two teaspoons of food is quite adequate in the first instance. Once you have discovered which foods the baby likes then the quantity can be increased. If the baby does not like the taste of a particular food do not force it to eat, the food can be re-introduced at a later date when the child has got used to a wider variety of foods. Around 6 months of age the baby will start to chew, although they will have no teeth at this stage. During the next 3 months the baby is able to move from puréed food to food with lumps. This is a good time to introduce finger foods such as a piece of carrot, a crust of bread or a rusk. Never leave a baby alone with finger foods as they could break off a chunk of food and this could choke them. When large chunks do break off it is safest to remove these from the baby. As the baby becomes more involved with the process of eating solid food so they will want to feed themselves. This is a good time to give them a spoon of their own and they can start to learn to feed themselves. Between the age of 5–8 months the baby will learn to drink from a cup (or feeder cup) and this will cut out the necessity for bottle or breast feeds. As the baby eats a larger variety and larger amounts of solid food so the intake of milk feeds can be cut down. By the end of the first year the baby may only be having a milk feed before going to bed in the evening. Sucking is a comforting and pleasurable experience for babies and they may be resistant to losing this altogether. Mealtimes should be a happy, pleasant experience for the baby and plenty of time should be given to enable the baby to learn to feed by themselves. However, this can also be a very messy process, so the baby's clothes and the area around the high chair needs to be well protected.

CARE OF BABIES

Nappy Changing

In most western countries, mothers will have a choice of which type of nappy they will use on their baby. There is a wide choice of disposable nappies available on the market which includes nappies designed to fit the size and gender of the baby. Disposable nappies can be expensive, but in calculating the expense a mother needs to take into consideration the cost of washing and drying terry towelling nappies. There is a wide choice in terry towelling nappies which come in different qualities, thicknesses and at differing prices. For families that have modern washing machines there is no problem in dealing with with laundering of terry towelling nappies; however, for the family without a washing machine, disposable nappies may be the most practical solution. Some mothers may choose to use towelling nappies for most of the time and only use disposable nappies when they take the baby away from home. Mothers who know that they intend to have a large family may opt for high quality terry towelling nappies as these will last through a number of children. The decision of which type of nappy to choose will depend upon the mother's preference and her domestic situation. A baby will need to be changed on average about six times a day, so in one week a baby will need about 50 disposable nappies or alternatively two dozen terry towelling nappies (to allow for washing and drying between use). A baby should not be left in a soiled or wet nappy for lengthy periods of time as this will not only be uncomfortable but will cause nappy rash.

Using terry towelling nappies

Terry towelling nappies need to be cleaned, sterilized and washed in boiling water between each usage. They also need to be thoroughly dried and aired before they are re-used. On removing a soiled or wet terry towelling nappy it first needs to be sluiced in a bucket of cold water, rinsed and placed in a lidded bucket containing water and a chemical sterilizing agent such as Napisan. The nappy is left in the sterilizing solution for the period of time recommended in the manufacturer's instructions. Once they have been sterilized they can be washed in a washing machine using the hottest cycle. Non-biological washing powder must be used as any other type of powder is likely to cause rashes or allergies to the baby's skin. They must always be thoroughly rinsed using the full rinse cycle on the machine. Adding a fabric conditioner which is suitable for sensitive skins to the rinse cycle will keep the nappies fluffy and soft.

There are a number of ways of folding terry towelling nappies so that they fit the baby properly and offer the fullest amount of protection in the right places. Only safety nappy pins must be used to secure the nappy as these have a special mechanism which prevents them from coming open by themselves. If terry towelling nappies are used then plastic pants will need to be put over the nappy to prevent bedding and clothing getting soiled. Wherever possible it is better for the baby's skin if plastic pants can be left off for periods of time (particularly during the night) to let the air circulate around the nappy and help the prevention of nappy rash. Plastic pants will need to be sterilized and washed in the same way as nappies.

Changing a nappy

In the home or the nursery there should be a specific area where the baby is changed. In this area there needs to be a trolley or shelf which contains all the things needed to change a baby, buckets or bins in which to place the soiled nappies, access to hot and cold water and a table or shelf which is large enough to accommodate a baby changing mat. If there is not a changing area available then before changing the baby it will be necessary to gather together all the things that you will need, for example:

◆ Changing mat
◆ Warm water in a bowl
◆ Cotton wool balls or baby wet wipes
◆ Barrier cream such as zinc and castor oil
◆ Toilct roll or tissues
◆ Clean nappy (if terry towelling you will also need plastic pants)
◆ Container for the soiled nappy

Lie the baby on the changing mat and undo or remove any clothing in order to get access to the nappy. **Remember, a baby must never, ever be left alone on a changing mat that is above floor level.**

Undo the nappy fastening, hold the baby's ankles together and lift the baby's bottom, remove the nappy and place in a bucket or

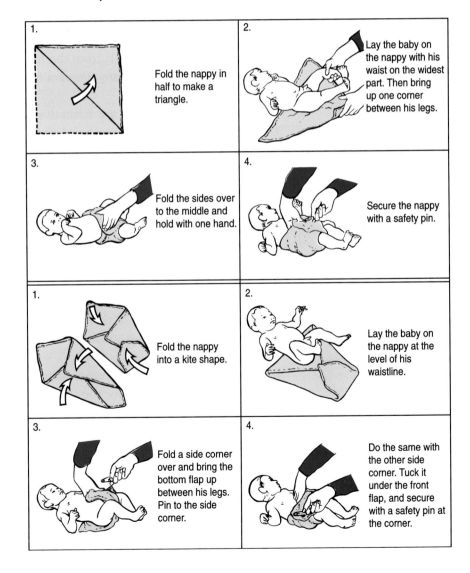

1. Fold the nappy in half to make a triangle.

2. Lay the baby on the nappy with his waist on the widest part. Then bring up one corner between his legs.

3. Fold the sides over to the middle and hold with one hand.

4. Secure the nappy with a safety pin.

1. Fold the nappy into a kite shape.

2. Lay the baby on the nappy at the level of his waistline.

3. Fold a side corner over and bring the bottom flap up between his legs. Pin to the side corner.

4. Do the same with the other side corner. Tuck it under the front flap, and secure with a safety pin at the corner.

Two ways of folding a terry towelling nappy.

other receptacle. Clean any faecal material with toilet roll. Using moist cotton wool or baby wipe clean the genital area first and then clean backwards towards the buttocks. Make sure that all faecal material or urine is removed. Dry the area thoroughly and apply the barrier cream. Put on the clean nappy and secure it. Put the baby in a safe place and then wash your hands.

Babies will usually need changing following a feed and this should be part of the routine care. They will also need checking at other regular intervals during the day to ensure that they do not have a wet or soiled nappy. Some babies do not like lying in a soiled or wet nappy and will let you know about this by crying until they are changed.

Nappy rash (see Chapter 2)

A common cause of nappy rash in the first month of life is thrush. This is an infection caused by a fungus which lives in warm moist areas such as mouth, intestines or vagina. It is common for newborn babies to become infected with this from the mother's birth canal. It is easily treated by getting an anti-fungal cream from the doctor.

Bathing a Baby

In most situations, babies are bathed using a baby bath; however, a baby can be bathed in a large bowl or in a large sink. The baby bath should be on a purpose-made stand or placed on a secure table or other flat surface. There are baby baths which fit into the adult bath or across the top of the adult bath. Whatever receptacle is used for bathing the baby it is important that it is on a secure surface where it cannot tip over and in a position that is easily reached by the person carrying out the bathing. Before bathing the baby all the equipment that will be needed should be placed within easy reach of the bath. All toiletries such as soap, talcum powder, shampoo, skin lotions and creams should be of a type that is suitable for babies or sensitive skin. There are a large number of these products on the market and they are all hypo-allergenic and so suitable for use on baby skin. In addition to the above items you will also need a small bowl of boiled water that has been left to cool, cotton wool balls, clean nappy, clean clothes, a warm towel, and a bucket for the soiled nappy and dirty clothes. Once all these items have been gathered together, fill the bath two-thirds full (remembering to put the cold water in first) of warm water. Test the temperature of the water by dipping your elbow into the water; it should be comfortably warm but not hot.

It is important during the whole process of bathing that the baby is held firmly so that it feels secure. The baby should be undressed on a changing mat or on your lap lying on a towel. Remove all the baby's clothes except the nappy and wrap him/her in the warm towel. Wash the baby's face with cotton wool moistened in the cooled boiled water. With moist cotton wool clean the area around the eyes using a clean piece of cotton wool for each eye. Holding the baby securely, hold his/her head over the bath and with your free hand wet the head, shampoo the scalp and then rinse away all traces of soap and dry with a towel. Do not be afraid to wash the fontanelle (soft spot) on top of the baby's head. Remove the baby's nappy, clean the bottom with damp cotton wool. Lower the baby into the bath whilst keeping your

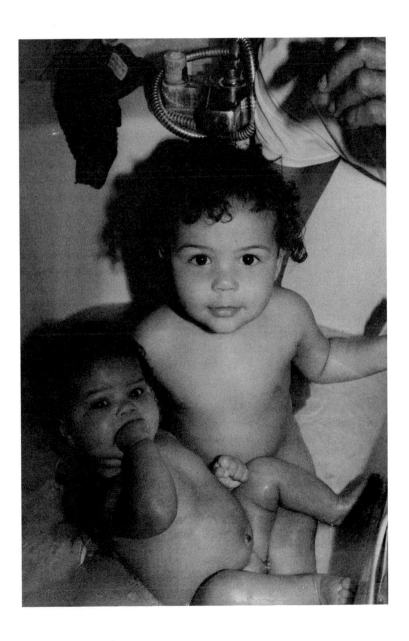

arm securely around him/her for support. Never let go of the baby when he/she is in the bath. Wash the baby thoroughly whilst giving him/her time to kick and splash in the water. Talk to the baby while you are bathing him/her as bath time should be an enjoyable experience in which the whole family can participate. Lift the baby out of the bath and wrap in a warm towel. Pat the baby dry and apply any necessary creams or lotions. Put on a clean nappy, clean clothes and place him/her somewhere safe whilst you tidy away the bath equipment.

Reducing the Risk of Cot Death

Cot death or sudden infant death syndrome (SIDS) is the term used to describe a baby that dies from no identifiable cause. In the UK it is the commonest cause of death in children under 1 year of age. Recent research has shown that there are precautions which can be taken to reduce the risk of cot death. Sadly, there is no advice which will guarantee that a baby will not die, but taking the precautions will lessen the risk. The Department of Health and the Foundation for the Study of Infant Deaths advise the following:

◆ Place the baby on the back or side to sleep
◆ Don't smoke and avoid placing the baby in smoky atmospheres
◆ Do not let the baby get too hot
◆ If you think the baby is unwell contact the doctor

If placing the baby on its side to sleep ensure that the underneath arm is brought forward in front of the body to prevent the baby rolling on to its tummy.

Babies that are exposed to tobacco smoke in the air they breathe are also at greater risk of cot death.

Babies do not need hot rooms. The ideal room temperature is 18°C (65°F). Babies lose excess heat from their heads so when putting them to bed do not cover their heads with bedclothes, hoods, hats etc. When bringing a baby from the outdoors into a warm room remember to remove the extra clothing as soon as you come inside. Duvets should not be used as bedclothes for babies under 1 year of age and bedclothes should be made of natural fibres, preferably cotton.

It is also recommended that a cot is made up so that babies sleep 'feet to foot', in other words, the baby's feet are at the foot of the cot and the blankets only cover the length of the baby. This reduces the risk of the baby getting their head under the blankets and being unable to regulate heat loss through the head. Parents and carers are advised to watch the press for any updated advice on the precautions relating to cot death as research into the subject is constantly being undertaken. As a result of the most recent research findings the above advice is the latest being publicized by the Department of Health and the Foundation for the Study of Infant Deaths (FSID) (this is the most current at the time of going to press); however, this may alter as new research findings are published.

Sleep Patterns of Babies

Not all babies will develop the same sleep patterns but most will settle into some type of routine during the first month. During the first year, babies are likely to sleep on average 14–16 hours per day. Half the sleeping time will be during the night and the remainder during the day. When babies sleep they divide the sleeping time into blocks of 2–3 hours with a wakeful period in between each block. As Kakar (1981) points out, putting children down to sleep at a regular time is a very 'western' idea. In Indian culture a child will 'sleep when it sleeps, wake up when it wakes up'. However, when parents work, where there is no extended family to help out, it is easier to get the child into a sleep routine that fits in with the routine of the parents and this can be achieved by putting children down to sleep at regular intervals during the day.

In order to promote sleep the baby needs to be in a comfortable environment, wearing comfortable clothes, not overwrapped or too hot, preferably recently fed and changed. The baby should be put somewhere quiet to sleep as loud noises will waken them.

Sleep and rest are necessary to promote the functioning of the circulatory and respiratory systems, give the brain and nervous system a chance to rest, prevent fretfulness and irritability, and generally helps the rebuilding of energy in the body.

Stimulating Babies

All babies need stimulation in order to develop intellectually, physically, socially, emotionally and linguistically. Babies develop at their own pace, and the rate of development may be dependent upon the amount and type of stimulation they are given. Different families and different lifestyles will offer different types of stimulation, for example, babies carried in slings will have a very different view of the world than a baby who is in a pram; babies in hot climates are able to benefit from an outdoor lifestyle which offers them a very different experience of movement and space compared with the baby that grows up in a high rise flat. Developmental scales and charts must therefore be used only as a guide and never viewed as 'tablets of stone' as it is unlikely that there is any baby that develops at a rate 'according to the charts'.

Jean Piaget in 1953 described the early stages of children's cognitive development as the sensorimotor period. This is a very apt description, as this is the period when the child learns through use of their senses and fine and gross motor movements (Bee, 1992). Evans (1978) writing about the HighScope system describes the first year of life in a different way:

the heads up stage (0–1 month)
the looker stage (1–4 months)
the creeper crawler stage (4–8 months)
the walker stage (8–12 months)
The ages are approximate as each child will grow at his/her own rate and some traits will stand out more than others.

There are numerous books available on child development which go into each stage in great detail. In the confines of this chapter it is only possible to take a cursory look at development and this has been done specifically in relation to examples of some of the ways in which babies can be stimulated during the first year of life. Opportunities to stimulate babies should not be lost or overlooked. The daily routine offers times when there is a one-to-one relationship between the child and the adult, for example, changing, bathing, feeding and dressing; all of these times offer good opportunities for the adult to talk to the baby and play with the baby. The baby will soon come to recognize the voices of the different adults that care for them. Around 1–2 months the baby will respond to the sound of

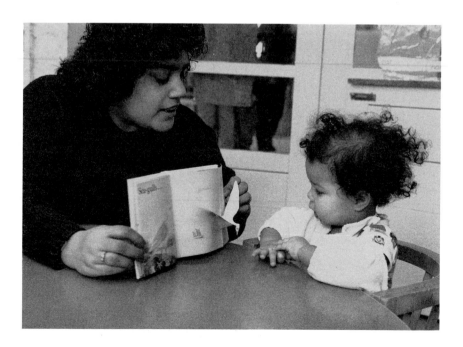

the adult's voice by trying to communicate with cooing and repeated vowel sounds.

It is not necessary to buy lots of toys in order to stimulate the baby. Mobiles, stuffed toys, balls etc. can be homemade or, at a later stage in their development, wooden spoons, saucepans and empty cardboard boxes all provide useful items for babies to explore. However, it is important to enure that any commercially bought toys have the British Standard Safety Kitemark and are labelled as being safe to use with children aged 1 year and under.

In the first 3 months of life babies learn through their senses (sight, hearing, taste, touch, smell), therefore it is a good idea to provide stimulation through these senses. A mobile placed above the cot at a distance of 20–25 cm (8 inches) from the child's eyes will help the baby focus. If the mobile also has a noise, such as a bell, it will also stimulate the baby's hearing and offer an added interest. Between 2–4 months the baby will smile in response to a familiar face. The baby will be able to raise their head, reach for objects and is able to clasp and unclasp their hands. At this stage, in addition to the mobile, a rattle is useful as this can be placed in their hands. They will like objects of different colours and textures, and a baby mirror fixed at eye level outside the cot will attract their attention when they turn their head towards it. Babies at this stage of development do not have what psychologists refer to as 'object permanence'. This means that when the toy has gone from the baby's view the baby does not look for or reach for the toy but just forgets it. When the baby drops the rattle it is forgotten, as the old adage says, 'out of sight out of mind'.

Between 4–6 months the baby should have good back and head control and be able to sit up. Around this time they develop the ability to pick up objects. They will now need more space and encouragement to move about and this can be done by placing bright colourful objects near to them which they can reach out for and grasp. This is the time they like to sit/lie on a blanket on the floor and play with toys such as a rattle, brightly coloured soft balls, things that can be grasped and investigated such as textured balls, small cardboard boxes etc. It is to be remembered that at this stage babies use their mouths to explore objects, so all toys must be checked for safety. At this stage the baby is also exploring their own body and they like moving their arms and legs, particularly if this movement can also move a mobile or a rattle which will produce a sound. Bath time is also good fun and babies will quickly learn to kick and splash about in the water. Between 6–8 months the baby will be able to sit alone, turn towards sound and be able to transfer objects from hand to hand. It is around this time that

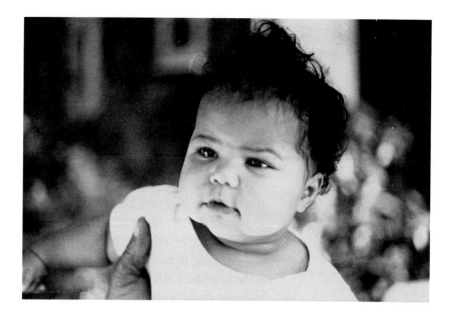

babies begin to develop object permanence. When they drop a toy from their high chair or cot they will look over the edge to see where it has gone. Many children find this dropping of objects a very enjoyable game when there is an adult present to pick them up! At this stage they are beginning to explore the world around them so they will need plenty of space to move around. Balls, stacking or nesting toys, large bricks and blocks are very useful for developing movement and enabling the baby to learn about space. At this stage babies will start to enjoy nursery rhymes that are active and repetitive, for example, 'Incy Wincy Spider', 'Round and Round the Garden' and 'Pat-a-Cake'. They will babble using consonants and vowel sounds trying out new sound patterns. They will have good hand to mouth co-ordination and will use the mouth to explore objects and even furniture.

Around 8–10 months the baby will reach the crawling/creeping stage and will try to pull themselves into a standing position. It is the time when special care needs to be taken to make sure that they are in a safe environment; particular attention should be paid to furniture as this needs to be stable and the corners of tables and chairs covered with soft protectors (these can be obtained from baby supply shops such as Mothercare). At this stage they will like to play games such as 'peek-a-boo' and games where they are shown a favourite object and it is then hidden from their sight and then revealed. Brightly coloured simple picture books will also be attractive to them, particularly those that contain familiar objects which can be named by the adult and the baby then has the opportunity to try to say the word. At this stage they will enjoy playing with household implements such as saucepans, wooden spoons, measuring spoons, a plastic jug etc.

At around 10–12 months they will probably be able to stand by themselves, will be able to use a spoon and can say their first words. This is also the time when they are exploring everything around them and extra safety precautions need to be taken; safety locks on cupboards, refrigerators and freezers, gates on kitchen doors and at the foot of stairs, all help to cut down the risks of accidents. A sturdy babywalker or push-along toy will encourage them to take their first steps whilst still being able to hold on for support. They will soon learn to push the walker towards a toy or other object that they are trying to reach. Activity centres, musical instruments such as a xylophone or shakers, bells, building materials such as wooden bricks, and cardboard boxes (particularly very large ones which they can crawl inside) help develop the child's skills whilst making it fun to learn.

Elinor Goldschmeid is the pioneer of the 'treasure basket' and 'heuristic play' for under-2-year-olds. The word heuristic comes from the Greek word *eurisko* which means 'to discover or reach an understanding of'. Heuristic play is provided by enabling babies to explore natural objects through the medium of a treasure basket. The treasure basket is a bag or basket containing a number of everyday natural objects which the child can explore and in doing so discover the properties of these objects. For heuristic play there is a need to have the same object in different sizes, objects which stack, objects of different colours and weights. For the under-1-year-olds, who will be finding out the very basic attributes of simple objects, a treasure basket containing a number of different objects is sufficient. The types of objects that can go in a treasure basket are as follows:

Natural objects:
Fir cones, shells, big feathers, corks, avocado pear stone, pumice stone etc.
Objects of natural materials:
Woollen ball, small shoe brush, bone ring, shaving brush, small raffia mat etc.
Wooden objects:
Small boxes, castanets, napkin ring, clothes pegs, egg cup, cotton reel etc.
Metal objects:
Spoons, bunch of keys, tea strainer, metal beaker, small tins, bunch of bells, bicycle bell etc.

Objects in leather, textile, rubber, fur:
Small teddy bear, fur ball, leather purse, velvet powder puff,
coloured marble eggs, bath plug and chain, etc.
Paper and cardboard objects:
Greaseproof paper, tinfoil, small cardboard boxes etc.

(Goldschmeid, 1989)

The main purpose of the objects in the treasure basket is to offer stimulus to the child's senses, and Goldschmeid states that it is for this reason that plastic items are not included in the objects as they have little stimulus to offer. It must not be forgotten that any objects in a treasure basket are likely to be put into the child's mouth so they must not be small enough for the child to swallow or dangerous in design or toxic. The child can then put their hand in the basket and each object will teach them something about shape, size, colour, hardness, softness and texture (rough, smooth etc.). Offering smaller baskets will enable the child to manipulate the objects and move them from place to place. The adult has the role of facilitator by collecting the objects together and making them available to the child. When the child is playing they can observe what the child does and which objects interest the child most. Even very young children will spend long periods of concentration playing with the objects in a treasure basket.

Parental Involvement

It is important that the child care worker responsible for the baby works with the parents so that the child has the best possible care; shared care is the best practice. Many parents lack confidence in dealing with their child, particularly if it is a first baby, and will be looking for reassurance from the childminder or child care worker. Ante-natal classes which concentrate on parent education would have given the parents some ideas as to how the baby will develop in the first few months of life. In the early days the midwife and health visitor will be available to advise and instruct. If a mother is lacking in confidence it is very useful to be able to put her in touch with other mothers. Organizations such as PIPPIN (Parent Infant Project) and Meet-a Mum provide a networking system between mothers with local group meetings and problem-solving skills for new parents (addresses at the back of the book).

It is important that when the parents develop a new skill they are encouraged and praised by the child care worker. It is very easy for the child care worker to take over completely and make the parents feel useless and de-skilled. The parents have to cope in the evenings and at weekends and it is important for the continuity of the child's care for the parents to know exactly how to handle their child in the very numerous situations which may arise. If the child care worker learns a new technique which encourages the child to do something better then this should be shared with the parents, likewise, if the child reaches a particular developmental stage when they are with the child care worker then the parents need to be informed that the baby can now drink from a cup, sit up, roll over etc.

Assignments

1. Describe how you would prepare a bottle feed for a 2-month-old baby.

2. 'Breast milk is best.' Discuss this statement.

3. Write the menus for a week for an 8-month-old baby who is partially weaned and only has a bottle feed before going to bed at night.

4. What is 'sudden infant death syndrome' and what precautions can be taken to lower the risk of this happening?

5. Describe how you would bath a 6-month-old baby.

6. What is heuristic play? What type of activities could you offer to a 1-year-old to develop this type of play?

7. What do you understand by the term 'shared care'? Why is it important to promote 'shared care'?

REFERENCES AND FURTHER READING

Bee, Helen (1992). *The Developing Child*, 6th edition. Harper Collins, New York.

Bowlby, John (1953). *Child Care and the Growth of Love*. Pelican, London.

Bowlby, John (1979). *The Making and Breaking of Affectional Bonds*. Tavistock, London.

Cowley, Liz (1994). *Young Children in Group Day Care: guidelines for good practice*, 2nd edition. National Children's Bureau, London.

Evans, J. (1978) *Good Beginnings*. HighScope Press, Ypsilanti, USA.

Goldschmeid, Elinor (1987). *Infants at Work (Notes)*. National Children's Bureau, London.

Goldschmeid, Elinor (1989). Play and learning in the first year of life. In *Babies in Daycare: An Examination of the Issues* (ed. Veronica Williams). The Daycare Trust, London.

Goldschmeid, Elinor (1990). What to do with under twos. Heuristic play. Infants learning. In *Babies and Toddlers: Carers and educators. Quality for the under threes*. National Children's Bureau, London.

Hilton, Tessa with Messenger, Maire (1993). *The Great Ormond Street Book of Baby and Child Care*. Bodley Head, London.

Jolly, Hugh (1986). *Book of Child Care*. Unwin Paperbacks, London.

Kakar, S (1981). *The Inner World – a psychoanalytic study of children and society in India*. Oxford University Press, Delhi.

Leach, Penelope (1988). *Baby and Child*. Penguin, London.

Pugh, Gillian, De'Ath, Erica and Smith, Celia (1994). *Confident Parents, Confident Children*. National Children's Bureau, London.

Reid, Joanna (1995). More than meets the eye (new research into babies). *Nursery World*, 23 November, p. 12.

Vincent Priya, Jacqueline (1992). *Birth Traditions and Modern Pregnancy Care*. Element, Dorset.

Williams, Veronica (ed.) (1989). *Babies in Daycare: an examination of the issues*. The Daycare Trust, London.

Chapter 6

Child Development

This chapter covers underpinning knowledge for all NVQs or courses in child care, including the CACHE Diploma and Certificate.
Whilst it is not linked with specific units or modules the material in this chapter underpins all work with children

INTRODUCTION

Child development is the study of how children develop as they grow physically, intellectually, linguistically, emotionally and socially (the well-known mnemonic (memory aid) for this being PILES). Whilst all human beings follow the same developmental pattern or order of development, there is great variety in individual performance. In other words children develop at different rates according to their environment, their abilities, the stimulation they receive and the opportunities that they are given to learn new skills. An understanding of child development is a very important part of the underpinning knowledge required by parents and child care workers. Having a knowledge of child development enables parents and carers to offer children the relevant experiences in order to aid the child's developmental progress.

The development of children is dependent upon a number of factors; however, the academics and researchers who produce theories on child development are often specialists in only one field and therefore study one area of development in depth. A study undertaken in this way may be in isolation from the other factors that are involved. Taken at its most literal, a knowledge of child development can be a very dangerous tool if it is used without thought or reference to all the factors which may have an effect upon it. It is important to always look at the child as a whole (the holistic view) and to take into consideration social and cultural factors.

For convenience, child development is written in a form that detracts from the holistic view of the child. It must therefore be remembered that each aspect of development is like a piece of a jigsaw puzzle which may be interesting in itself but only makes sense when it is part of the whole picture. For example if a child is feeling unwell (physical) they will not want to participate in learning activities or play (intellectual), they may be fretful and irritable (emotional) and may not respond to attempts to include them in interaction with their parents or carers or others (social), and they may revert to baby talk to explain their symptoms (linguistic).

A good method of studying child development is by observing children and this is why most child care courses place a great emphasis on child observations. Many students begin to learn the skill of observing by watching videos of children in different stages of development; following this they progress to carrying out observations when they are in practical work placements. With a knowledge of child development theories a student can then evaluate the observation. There are a large number of books devoted just to child development and some of these can be found in the reference section at the end of this chapter. Suffice to say that it is impossible to give more than a brief outline of development within the confines of this chapter. It needs to be remembered that there is not one single child development theorist who is accepted by all the experts; most people use parts from a number of theorists.

In describing aspects of child development, writers use terms such as 'norm', 'milestones', 'approximate ages', 'stages' etc. in order to produce a set of benchmarks along the development continuum. It is necessary for writers to do this in order to transfer ideas and theories in a way which can be understood by their readers. All children develop at their own pace and there is unlikely to be in existence a 'normal' child that reaches all the milestones at the target ages as laid down in the literature.

CULTURAL ASPECTS OF CHILD DEVELOPMENT

Cassie Landers (1995) describes culture as

> a body of learned meaning and shared information transmitted from generation to generation through interaction ... therefore cultural variations in child rearing influence children's mental, emotional and social development, just as such variations determine which language a child will eventually speak. Parental approaches to child-rearing in different cultures are similar in some ways but different in others.

This broad definition of culture put forward by Landers (1995) enables those involved with child development to take culture into account in its widest sense. In other words, culture encompasses class, race, ethnicity, environment, religion, politics, gender, and anything else which may contribute towards the way in which a family group forms its value system. It is these values which are then passed on from

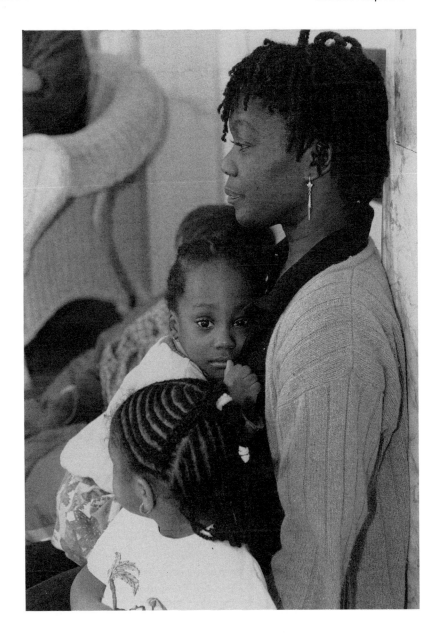

generation to generation. Such values will influence the way parents/carers approach child rearing and view child development. For example, environmental issues such as climate will influence the culture. Hot countries have an outdoor culture, whereas cold/temperate countries will have an indoor culture. Children living in hot countries are likely to have more freedom in terms of space and this in turn may lead to them having earlier developmental patterns in gross motor movements such as walking, running, jumping, climbing etc.

Families and individuals are able to accept or reject these shared values which are continually being updated and refashioned. When studying child development it needs to be remembered that parents/family will interpret the world to the child and this interpretation will be influenced by how the adults see the world (cultural influences). It is also necessary for child care workers to consider how their own value systems/culture influence the ways in which they deal with children and their parents/carers.

CHILD DEVELOPMENT THEORISTS

As already stated there is not one theorist who satisfies all the experts in the field; however, it might be useful to have some knowledge of the most well known.

Piaget

This Swiss biologist and psychologist is a central figure in the school of cognitive development theory. Piaget's theories, which were based upon many years of research and observation of children, outlined stages of intellectual development (see Table 6.1).

Table 6.1 Piaget's stages of intellectual development

Stage	Approximate ages
1. *Sensorimotor period*	Birth to 2 years
Sub-stage I	Birth to 1 month
Sub-stage II	1–4 months
Sub-stage III	4–10 months
Sub-stage IV	10–12 months
Sub-stage V	12–18 months
Sub-stage VI	18 months to 2 years
2. *Pre-operational thought period*	2–7 years
Preconceptual phase	2–4 years
Intuitive phase	4–7 years
3. *Period of concrete operations*	7–11 years
4. *Period of formal operations*	11–15 years

Piaget's work shows that before a child can progress from one stage to another, both maturation (internal growth) and appropriate learning must take place. Special training to try to enhance/speed up this process is only temporarily effective and the child tends to revert to their natural developmental level. Piaget showed that intellectual development is not simply an accumulation of changes but is a process whereby the child constructs their own understanding of self, others and the world around them. In order to do this the child is consistently trying to adapt to the world around them, which leads them to pass through stages of increasing complexity of thought. Piaget called these stages sensorimotor, pre-operational thought, concrete operations and formal operations. Piaget states that there is a constant interaction between emotional and intellectual aspects of development so that in times of stress a child may regress to an earlier level of thinking. Emotional difficulties can prevent progression to the next level of thinking and may render the person to never be able to reach full logical functioning.

There has been criticism of Piaget's theories on the grounds that he seems to have been wrong about the way in which cognitive skills develop. Work by Susan Martorano (1977) has shown that a child may perform at one stage on one task and at another stage on a second task even though the two tasks seem to require the same basic cognitive thought.

Freud

Freud was the founder of a school of thought known as psychoanalysis which states that the development of the child's personality is greatly influenced by the child's relationship with its parents. According to Freud the infant's relationship with its mother develops as a secondary consequence of the way she provides relief from hunger and thirst. The child develops emotional dependence upon the mother by its own efforts to reduce the discomfort of hunger and thirst. Freud maintained that the child's developmental progress could be seen in psychosexual stages (see Table 6.2). The stages are characterized by certain sources of sexual gratification.

Table 6.2 Freud's stages of psychosexual development

Stage	Approximate age	Characteristics
Oral	0–8 months	Sources of pleasure include sucking, biting, swallowing, playing with lips; pre-occupation with immediate gratification of impulses
Anal	8–18 months	Sources of sexual gratification include expelling faeces and urinating, as well as retaining faeces
Phallic	18 months to 6 years	Child becomes concerned with genitals; source of sexual pleasure involves manipulating genitals; period of Oedipus or Electra complex
Latency	6–11 years	Loss of interest in sexual gratification; identification with same-sexed parent

Erikson

Erikson, a psychologist, looked primarily at social development of children. Erikson's theory puts forward eight developmental stages (the first four are described in Table 6.3). Erikson's stages of development cover the whole lifespan, not just the period of childhood. The eight stages are as follows.

1. Basic trust versus basic mistrust
2. Autonomy versus shame, doubt
3. Initiative versus guilt
4. Industry versus inferiority
5. Identity versus role confusion
6. Intimacy versus isolation
7. Generativity versus stagnation
8. Ego integrity versus despair

Table 6.3 Erikson's development phases, 0–9 years

Approximate ages	Psychosocial crises	Radius of significant relations	Psychosocial modalities	Psychosexual stages
0–8 months	1 Trust versus mistrust	Maternal person	To get: to give in and return	Oral-respiratory sensory-kinesthetic
8–18 months	2 Autonomy versus shame and doubt	Parental persons	To hold on: to let go	Anal-urethral, muscular - (retentive-eliminative)
18 months to 6 years	3 Initiative versus guilt	Basic family	To make (going after): to make like (playing)	Infantile-genital locomotor
6–9 years	4 Industry versus inferiority	Neighbourhood, school	To make things (completing): to make things together	Latency

Erikson's theory argues that the presence of conflict stemming from the person's need to adapt to a social environment produces certain types of thinking. Resolution of the conflict results in the development of a new competence. Erikson sees the first characteristic of infancy as 'trust versus mistrust', that is a natural mistrust of the world about which the child knows nothing and yet there is a need to arrive at feelings of security and trust. Although confrontation and resolution of this and other conflicts continues throughout life, the safe and reliable environment provided for the child helps them to overcome the early mistrust. As does Freud, Erikson believes that the basic mistrust centres around bodily functions such as eating and emotions associated with these functions.

The differences between Freud and Erikson are that Freud maintains that all the cognitive skills develop only because the child needs them to obtain gratification whereas Erikson maintains that the ego functions are presumed to develop independently even though they are used to obtain basic gratification. For a more fuller explanation of these theories see Bee (1992, chapter 7).

Bandura

Bandura is a social learning theorist who looks primarily at the reinforcement patterns in the environment as being responsible for the differences in children's behaviour patterns. Whilst accepting biological factors such as hormones and inherited characteristics do have a role to play in forming a child's behaviour pattern, Bandura maintains that the greatest influences are the environmental factors. For example, a child care worker who only pays attention to children when they are noisy and rowdy will be reinforcing this type of behaviour pattern and therefore the children will become more rowdy and noisy in order to gain attention. Bandura's theories are the basis for many positive reinforcement programmes which are used with children who exhibit extreme behaviours.

Bruner

Bruner's developmental theories have been influenced by the work of Piaget as they both believe that children are born with a biological organization which enables them to understand the world around them, and as their cognitive structures mature so they can think in an ever more complex way, and that children have an innate curiosity which enables them to explore and adapt to their environment through interaction with it. However, Bruner's theory is not about stages of development but is three ways of representing the world, enactive, iconic and symbolic, and children develop them in that order. Enactive is representation of the world through actions and what has been experienced through a baby's own behaviour. Iconic is when the child builds up a mental image of things they have experienced. Symbolic is the change that occurs around 6–7 years of age and is when language has an influence on thought.

STAGES OF DEVELOPMENT

For other details of development in the first year see Chapter 5.

1–3 Months

Physical development

The newborn baby is endowed with primitive reflex actions, which are responses to stimuli. The earliest and most essential reflex is that of sucking. When placed with their cheek next to the breast the baby roots around until they find the nipple which they then suck. This is a primitive reflex to satisfy the basic need for food. At 1 month the child begins to associate sucking with satisfaction and comfort and this reflex becomes a voluntary action. Most reflexes disappear within 4 weeks of birth.

At 1 month the baby has lost some of the neonatal reflex actions but will still make reflex walking actions if held standing on a hard surface. If the cheek is touched the baby will turn their head to one side. The baby's head falls forward if they are held in a sitting position to form a C curve with the rest of the body. Grasping, rooting and random movements are present in the first month.

At 3 months the baby shows anticipatory actions by moving arms and legs. The grasp reflex, which is lost by the age of 3 months, is when an adult finger is placed on the palm of each hand the newborn baby will respond by grasping so tightly that the baby can be pulled up from the lying position. If a piece of rope is grasped by the baby and suspended above the cot the baby will hang without danger of falling, such is the strength of the grasping reflex. These early reflexes are seen as precursors to later stages in development such as holding objects and walking. When the baby hears a sudden loud noise the baby responds with the startle reflex. The arms are flung outwards and then brought in towards the body. Another reflex which is useful is the ability to turn the head to one side when the baby is placed on their back.

Intellectual development

At 1 month of age the baby responds to stimuli of light and movement. They turn their head and eyes towards the light and can follow a pencil light for a little while when it is held about 30 cm (12 inches) away from them. When the light is shone directly at them the baby will shut their eyes tight, a defence mechanism which persists through life. If a dangling toy or rattle is shaken about 15–20 cm (6–8 inches) away from the baby's eyes they will follow it as it is moved from side to side. Experiments have shown that babies respond not only to human faces but to drawings resembling human faces. At 1 month the baby watches the mother's face as they feed.

Feeding presents valuable opportunities for learning and in breast feeding the baby explores taste, smell and touch. It is thought that the senses of touch, taste and smell are more acute at birth. The baby's heightened sensitivity to smell is shown in their ability to distinguish between the smell of breast milk and sugar water.

Helping the child's intellectual development in the first 3 months involves extending the stimulation provided in everyday activities of feeding, bathing and changing nappies. Babies should be spoken to from birth as this aids development of language and acts as auditory stimulation. Adequate stimulation is essential for all aspects of development: babies left in cots gazing up at white walls and ceilings, deprived of interaction with adults show all the signs of failing to thrive. In studies undertaken on the long term effects of stimulation in babies it was discovered that babies who had not been stimulated did not learn new tasks as quickly as those who had the right amount of stimulation. However, over-stimulation does not accelerate development; hanging numerous mobiles above a cot, having highly coloured and patterned wallpaper and flowery cot sheets would present over-stimulation and would be likely to cause the baby distress. Thus the right balance needs to be achieved.

A single colourful mobile (which could be homemade) suspended above the cot is sufficient for the first 2–3 months. After this period a more complex shape could be used. Mobiles need to be brightly coloured in order to gain the child's attention. At 1 month the child will simply lie and look at it; at 2 months they will attempt to hit it, but without success as they have not yet achieved eye/hand co-ordination to enable them to make direct contact with the object. Such complex co-ordination does not develop until around 5 months of age.

Language development

Babbling often begins around 2 months of age and is repeated 'play speech' rather than communication as the baby repeats sounds just for pleasure. Even babies with deaf parents will babble although their parents cannot hear or respond to them. While babbling is not essential to the development of speech it does provide verbal practice which lays the foundation for developing a recognizable language. It is a good idea for the adult to encourage babbling by repeating the sounds that the baby makes. This delights the baby who is encouraged to develop a range of noises.

Emotional development

The formation in early infancy of secure attachments with constant adults is crucial for the child's future emotional development. Security is a basic need as much as food, warmth and protection. A feeling of trust is essential for human relationships. Even at 1 month of age babies respond to a soothing voice and a cuddle. Anxiety or tension can easily be transmitted to the baby through rough handling or a short temper. A mother who is upset and worried and complains that the baby is always crying may not realize how her own emotional distress can upset the baby.

Most mothers tend to position their babies on their left side. This means that the baby can hear the mother's heart beating, and studies show that babies find this very soothing and reminiscent of their intrauterine life. It has also been discovered that babies whose mothers listened to music during pregnancy slept happily in the first months of life with a radio or record player on.

Social development

While the child's first relationship is usually with its parents, they are also able to form attachments with others, and it is the quality of the interaction (rather than the length) which appears to be the important factor. Whether the primary care-giver is the child's biological mother or not, there will exist from the earliest days a reciprocity of communication. The mother or primary care-giver is sensitive to the baby's signals – smiles, cries or babbling – and their response establishes early socialization as a partnership. The basis for communication is laid in the dialogue between care-giver and baby; the baby responds by imitating or offering another initiative. This important interaction is observed in all the mutual experiences shared by care-giver and baby – feeding, bathing, playing, nappy changing, bedtime – and serves to reinforce and develop the relationship. Thus as the baby learns about their social environment by initiating contact with and responding to their care-giver, the care-giver's interest in the baby increases and so furthers the partnership. At 5 weeks the baby may smile at their care-giver when they talk to the baby and at 6 weeks may 'talk back' by gurgling in response to the care-giver's voice. Observations of babies from birth to 1 month have shown that they will gaze for a longer period of time at the human face or drawings and cut-out images which resemble the face. By 6 weeks, most babies carry out detailed examination of the human face, with the eyes seeming to hold the greatest fascination.

3–6 Months

Physical development

At 3 months of age the baby can keep their head erect for a few seconds when held in the sitting position. This is due to bone and muscle development in the cervical region of the vertebral column; it also enables the baby to move their head to look around. The baby's limbs now move more easily and when placed on their tummy they are able to lift their head and upper trunk using their forearms for support. When held standing with their feet on a hard surface the legs will sag at the knees. At 3 months the reflex actions have usually disappeared and the baby has some voluntary movements which they like to repeat. Finger play involves clasping and unclasping hands and the baby likes to watch the movement of their hands. At 5 months the baby can reach out to grasp with both hands. One month later their range of abilities will be extended as they develop the palmar grasp which enables them to use the whole hand as a scoop, and soon they will be happy to use just one rather than both hands. At this stage everything is taken to the mouth as oral exploration is the main sensory activity.

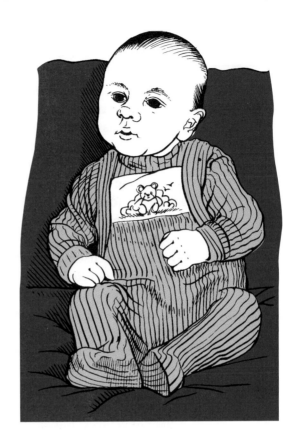

A baby of 6 months can sit upright with support.

Intellectual development

This stage is characterized by the beginnings of intentional activity in that the baby repeats actions in order to make interesting events last. If small bells are suspended across the cot and the baby discovers the bells will ring if a cord is pulled, they will continue to pull the cord, although not in the sense of using a stimulus to bring about a response as they are not yet old enough to link the activities; they simply want to make an interesting result persist, in the same way that they will repeatedly shake a rattle.

At this stage babies still think that when an object is out of sight it is no longer in existence, and when a toy falls out of their hand it is forgotten if it cannot be seen. At 4-6 months the baby will reach out to take a partially covered object but is unable to obtain an object that has been completely covered by a cloth as the object ceases to exist once it is out of sight. When a 5-month-old baby is presented with a stationary object that proceeds to move they can follow it wherever it goes. The child now seems able to realize that an object can go from place to place through movement, although their visual perception (or ability to translate and understand the information they receive through sight) seems to be ahead of their sensorimotor co-ordination.

Another result of the baby's playing is 'object attainment' which means that they come to appreciate that an object seen in different ways will still be the same object. Thus when the baby is able to hold the bottle and suck from the teat they will attempt to suck the bottom if the bottle is presented to them upside down. At a later stage, when they have come to recognize it is an enduring object, they will turn it round the right way before sucking.

During this period the baby is able to distinguish between simple geometric forms such as circles, squares and triangles. These can be used as mobiles, or plastic shapes can be given to the baby to grasp – provided they are large enough not to be swallowed! Familiarity with the three-dimensional shapes through sight, touch, taste and movement can be developed.

Language development

The 6-month-old baby provides a reward for the adult who has constantly persisted with the spoken word as the child vocalizes in single and double syllables which sound very like 'mum' and 'dada', and are eagerly translated as such by delighted parents. Familiar noises like that of the voice of the primary care-giver, preparation of feeds, running water in the bath etc. are greeted with laughs, chuckles and delighted squeals, but screams of annoyance fill the air if the baby's expectations are not fulfilled. The adult cannot ignore these overtures and responds with reinforcement of desired words. The baby quickly realizes that certain sounds provoke a pleased response from the adult and the baby provides their own reinforcement as they shout to attract attention. The baby also pauses to listen for the response and if it is not forthcoming, shouts again. The baby's powers of imitation are evident as they imitate the coughing, smacking of lips and other sounds that they hear around them.

Emotional development

A firm but gentle way of handling the baby contributes to feelings of security and trust and is particularly necessary for bath time when any hesitation on the adult's part can make the baby scream with terror. At 6 months the baby is clearly able to distinguish between different emotional tones in the voice of the primary care-giver. A quiet but not flat tone of voice, showing interest, care and even delight, will enhance the relationship with the child.

During the first 3 months, there are subtle, but no less definite, changes in the relationship between care-giver and child. These changes are partly due to the care-giver's growing self-confidence but also occur in response to the maturational changes in the baby. The baby is now awake more, cries less and spends more time smiling, vocalizing and looking at the care-giver's face. Meanwhile the care-giver is gradually decreasing the amount of very close physical contact, spends more time near the infant, increases affectionate behaviour, provides more stimulation and is more socially responsive towards the child.

Social development

As early as 3 months a baby recognizes the voice of its primary care-giver and shows delight in familiar happenings such as feeding, bathing and dressing, by smiling, cooing and moving their legs and arms. Studies with babies of 4–6 months of age reveal that the younger infants respond happily to multiple images of the care-giver whereas older babies become agitated as they realize that this is unnatural and prefer one stable image. They do not distinguish between strangers and familiars at this stage. Around 6 months, the baby may show anxiety or slight shyness in the presence of strangers – especially if the care-giver is out of sight. The presence of the primary care-giver acts as a pivot on which an enlarging circle of relationships turns. The child gains confidence from the security of firm but gentle handling and the satisfaction of expectations in basic need areas such as feeding.

6–9 Months

Physical development

The baby now holds their head erect with their back straight and although they may be able to sit up alone for a few seconds their back should still be well supported. The baby can raise their head and chest when placed face downwards, and is able to bear their own weight on their feet and bounce up and down when held in the standing position. At this age the baby uses their arm and wrist muscles to pull objects towards them and grasps them with the whole hand using the palmar grasp (eye–hand co-ordination). The baby has also discovered that their feet are useful playthings and may use them for grasping, although prefers to put them in their mouth! As the baby is able to sit up with support they will turn their head from side to side and their eyes will follow any movements of objects in their direct vicinity.

At 9 months the child's exploration of their environment involves movement of their trunk in rolling as a preliminary to crawling and standing with support. The child is very observant, manipulates objects by passing them from hand to hand and pokes them with their index finger. The baby can sit alone for up to 15 minutes (on the floor), turn their body sideways and move about by rolling on their tummy. The baby may also begin to crawl, although some children miss out this stage, preferring instead to shuffle along on their bottoms using one hand for support. They can stand holding on to a support for a few minutes, but cannot lower themselves to the sitting position. When the baby is held standing they take 'steps' on alternate feet and can stretch out for objects that they see in front of them. When they pick up items from the floor they use the finger and thumb in a scissor fashion and are less likely to put objects into their mouth. They will begin to explore objects by touch or visually or use the object for rhythmic banging.

Intellectual development

If the child is asked to hand over an object it may obey this instruction, but they do not offer objects voluntarily. Object attainment has now extended to a realization of object permanence – they appreciate that an object, though hidden from sight, still exists and will look under a cloth to find a toy. At this stage they enjoy games of 'peek-a-boo'. This involves temporarily hiding from the baby; providing the play partner reappears fairly soon, the baby can enjoy the game without feeling afraid. Often laughter is mingled with fear as the child feels insecure when someone leaves them all alone; as yet they cannot appreciate the notion of time or the meaning of temporary. The baby is now able to search in the correct place for the toys they have dropped within reach and will look after toys which have fallen from the pram or chair. The baby's newly developed understanding of object permanence and ability to direct activity towards an end (e.g. removal of a cover before the toy can be discovered) is, according to Piaget, the precursor of adult problem solving.

Bruner uses the term 'early play' to describe the range of activities enjoyed by the 6-month-old after they have learned to hold an object and get it easily to their mouth. 'Mastery play' is what Bruner calls the stage when the baby's actions with the object demonstrate their developing abilities. For example, first they look at the object, shake it, bang it on their chair, drop it over the edge and before long are able to fit the object into every possible activity. All this newly acquired mastery is applied to every new object, and Bruner found it surprising that at 6–8 months, babies can carry on such varied activities for as long as 30 minutes.

Emotional development

Around 7–8 months of age the child will show a natural anxiety, or 'fear of strangers'. This often upsets members of the wider family circle who are puzzled when the child begins to scream when they approach. However, if the primary carer or another adult that is very close to the child is present the fear can be easily resolved. This 'fear of strangers' combined with the ability to realize that unseen objects still exist (object permanence) explains the delight of the child in playing 'peek-a-boo' type games. Some minor fear can also be exciting. Like adults who love the thrill of fairground rides and enjoy screaming lustily to exhibit this fear, so babies scream with delight when a known face suddenly appears from behind a door or bobs up again in front of the pram. However, at this stage, the child will be distressed at any real separation from a familiar person.

Social development

At 9 months the use of hearing and speech in social development is evident as the baby uses babbling noises, loud noises, 'mmm', 'bah bah' and 'duh duh' sounds to attract attention and communicate. This is highly successful as parents and care-givers eagerly translate these meaningless sounds into 'mummy', 'daddy' and 'baby' and they naturally respond with more attention, reassurance and reinforcement of acceptable behaviour. As previously stated, at this stage the baby may respond negatively to strangers and will not accept them happily unless a familiar adult is present, although they may respond with a 'selective social smile'.

Signs of developmental delay at 5–8 months

Landers (1995) states that a baby who shows any of the following signs of developmental delay should be seen by a doctor or health visitor:

One or both eyes consistently turns in or out
Has difficulty getting objects to her mouth
Does not roll over in either direction by five months
Does not smile spontaneously by five months
Cannot sit without help by six months
Does not smile or make squealing sounds by six months
Does not actively reach for objects by six or seven months
Does not bear some weight on legs by six or seven months
Does not babble by eight months

(Landers, 1995)

9–12 Months

Physical development

Between 10–12 months the baby begins to pull themselves up to a standing position and can let themselves down while holding on to furniture. At 12 months they may try walking around a low table in a sideways fashion. Some babies can stand alone for a few minutes and even walk with one or both hands held by an adult. Other babies may not walk until they are 14–16 months of age, but this is just due to variation in the pace of development. The first movements which indicate that the baby is gaining voluntary control of the small muscles include the pincer grasp using thumb and index finger which the baby uses to pick up small toys and small pieces of food. At this stage they may be experimenting with feeding themselves, but the enormous opportunities for exploratory play with different foods and liquids often takes precedence over the necessity to actually eat, although if the child is really hungry the food will eventually find its way into their mouth.

Once they have been shown, the baby can click two blocks together or build a tower from two or three small blocks. Whilst most babies at this stage use both hands they may begin to show a preference for one hand; this is the beginning of right and left handedness. The baby can drink from a cup with a little help and can hold a spoon; however, they may have difficulty in using it properly without help. They are able to clap their hands in imitation of adults and also wave 'bye-bye'.

Exploration of the environment is extended by the baby's ability to crawl, which rapidly leads to standing whilst holding on to furniture, walking with one or both hands held by the adult, or stepping sideways around furniture. The baby's self-confidence increases with their ability to move around.

Intellectual development

Due to the baby's developing ability to co-ordinate movements it is possible to detect the means and the ends to their activities. They may grasp the bell by the handle and ring it in imitation of the adult; they are able to manipulate objects in the environment and will put wooden cubes into a cup or box and then lift them out again. To the baby's delight they may find that they are able to manipulate adults, as they drop toys deliberately and watch them fall to the ground, only to be picked up by whoever is passing by and returned to the baby who promptly drops them again! The repetitive action strengthens their sense of control over events and demonstrates the baby's understanding of 'object permanence' as they look in the correct place for the toy which has gone out of sight. They are able to point with their index finger and as already stated are able to use a pincer movement to pick up small objects. The baby's behaviour indicates that they are able to discriminate differences in people and things and they move from shyness and uneasiness with strangers to an acceptance, although they are still dependent upon their primary carer. The baby is able to begin to understand and perceive relationships between new and old situations and this is helped if the new material has something in common with past experiences. This is the beginning of coming to understand the world around them and the development of concepts which help them to order their understanding of the environment.

Language development

The baby is now able to recognize their own name and turns around in response to their name being called. The baby shows that they are able to understand simple commands accompanied by gestures, such as, 'Give me the spoon', 'Clap your hands'. The baby's self-confidence increases with their knowledge of their own name and the understanding of simple words relating to the world around them e.g. cup, spoon, walk, clap, dinner, ball, car etc. The adult is able to help the baby extend their language by continual repetition and explanation of day-to-day activities.

Emotional development

At this stage babies, as Penelope Leach (1988) points out, have strong emotions but have very little control over them. Their loves, hates, wishes and desires appear to be as strong as those of adults, but without language and physical mobility they are unable to do anything about them. This in itself leads to frustration and crying in situations

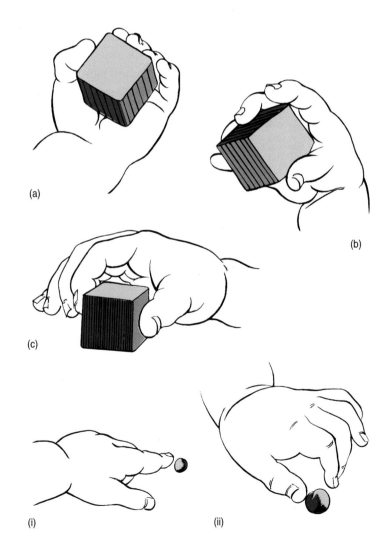

(a) Fine motor movements.
(b) Palmar grasp (6 months).
(c) Pincer grasp (12 months).
Then (i) pointing with index finger (9 months); (ii) picking up small objects (12 months).

which they cannot change. They will also cry at the unexpected, such as changes in routine, changes in the primary carer, going on a swing for the first time, first meeting with a large animal etc. At this stage, apart from hunger or illness, crying is a reaction to fear or an explosion of frustration and anger; the baby may need a comfort object such as a blanket, furry toy or even their thumb.

Social development

As the baby approaches the end of their first year they come to realize that adults can be used to provide help in play with objects and that objects can be used to gain the attention of adults.

Signs of developmental delay at 12 months

Landers (1995) states that if babies are exhibiting any of the following signs at 12 months of age then a doctor or health visitor should be consulted:

Drags one side of the body while crawling (existing for over one month)
Cannot stand when supported
Does not search for objects that are hidden while she watches
Says no single word (such as 'mama' or 'dada')
Does not learn to use gestures such as waving or shaking the head
Does not point to objects or pictures

(Landers, 1995)

15–18 Months

Physical development

At about 15 months the child can usually walk, but unsteadily and there may be frustrations and anger as they bump into furniture. They can also get to their feet alone, sit down backwards (with a bump), or fall forward onto their hands and then sit. They can crawl upstairs and therefore safety measures should include a stair gate which is strong, stable and able to withstand the child's weight. Leg muscles may be sufficiently developed to enable the child to bend and pick up toys from the floor. The child is able to hold a cup and bring a spoon to their mouth in order to lick it, but they may lack sufficient muscle control to hold it in one position for any length of time. At this stage large wheeled toys with handles which are very stable are useful as the child loves to push them and this helps them to practise walking by offering them support. Small muscle control can be seen in the way the child is able to pick up small objects and crumbs between the thumb and finger. Provided they are first shown how, the child is able to build a tower of two cubes and grasp a large crayon and scribble with it.

By 18 months the child should be able to walk well, start and stop safely, push and pull large toys and cardboard boxes around the floor

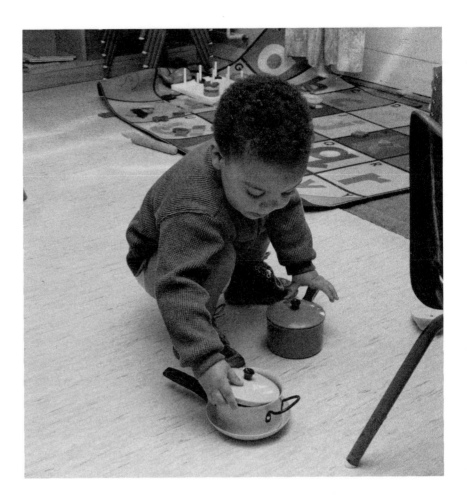

and carry a large bear or other soft toy whilst they are walking. They are able to run but in an awkward manner and they are able to stop in front of furniture. Whilst the child is able to sit down by leaning backwards into a small chair, they will usually climb forward into an adult-sized chair and then turn round in order to sit. Balance is now sufficiently controlled to enable the child to pick up toys from the floor without falling over. The child can walk upstairs with the aid of an adult and crawl downstairs backwards, although they may prefer bumping down on their bottom.

Fine motor movements involve spontaneous scribbling with a chunky pencil or crayon (and they may prefer to use one particular hand to do this), building a tower of three cubes, turning the pages of a book two or three at a time, pointing at pictures, holding a cup in

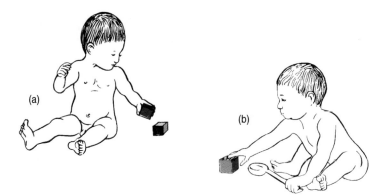

Small muscle control: (a) placing one cube on top of another (15 months); (b) arranging cubes horizontally (18 months).

both hands and drinking without excess spillage, using a spoon to get food into their mouth, and taking off their shoes, socks and hat.

Between 12–18 months the anterior fontanelle (which is the soft spot at the front of the skull) closes.

Intellectual development

The child shows an even greater curiosity and experimentation through trial and error with different objects by using different aspects of their sensorimotor development. For example, if the child is in the playpen, they may experiment with various movements or objects to bring a toy from its position outside through the bars. Thus they are demonstrating increasing control over their environment. Greater exploration is possible as they are now able to crawl upstairs and walk a few steps. Adult supervision is required to prevent possible dangers in this extended environment, but this should not be obstructive or hinder the child's curiosity. Valuables and ornaments should be kept out of reach as the child will explore everything they find. A large wheeled toy is popular as it aids their independence in walking, and picture books are appreciated as they offer visual stimulation.

The child will take pleasure in imitating adult expressions and actions. If shown how to scribble they will use a crayon and copy and by 18 months will spontaneously scribble. At 15 months the child is often able to indicate when they have soiled their nappy but is not yet neurologically mature enough to be toilet trained. Hand preference is becoming more marked and should not be discouraged or altered. Myths abound about the merits of being right-handed, as in the past it was seen to be a disadvantage to be left-handed. This may have originated from the Latin term for right, which is *dexter*, and people who are dexterous or have manual dexterity are admired within society. However, the Latin term for left is *sinister* and this has negative connotations within our society. However, research has shown that hand preference is associated with the side of the brain which is most dominant, therefore those who are right-handed have a left-brain dominance and those who are left-handed have a right-brain dominance. The research has not shown that there is any difference in the abilities of left-handed and right-handed people. In fact in racquet sports it is a distinct advantage to be left-handed!

Language development

By the age of 18 months the child will continuously talk to themselves in their own tuneful babble. They can use about 20 simple words but understand many more. They make their demands known by shouting, pointing or using simple words. The adult is able to help the child's language development by singing; reciting simple nursery rhymes which the child likes and will attempt to join in with; naming various parts of the baby (hair, nose, arm, foot) and encouraging the child's efforts to demonstrate their knowledge of where the part is. Simple picture books are enjoyed as the child is able to point out simple objects and the adult talks and tells a story about the objects.

Language is more than speech as it involves cognitive development. Piaget maintained that the development of certain logical concepts frequently precedes the understanding of words corresponding to those concepts. Words such as 'bigger', 'smaller', 'longer', 'further' are not understood until the logical properties themselves are understood by the child. Language and thinking have separate roots and develop independently. The evidence of thought before language in the pre-verbal child is unquestionable and this can also be seen in children with learning disabilities who are able to answer questions about the content of their reading by pointing out the written word answer, despite their inability to verbalize more than two or three words.

Emotional development

As the child struggles towards independence they are still emotionally vulnerable and require constant reassurance. At this stage they may develop an anxiety when they are put to bed at night and will want a favourite toy or comforter; it is also important to leave on a night-light if they develop a fear of the dark. They may become more clingy and want to be at the primary carer's side all the time, or they may worry about strange places and new faces.

Social development

This is the stage just before temper tantrums when the child is striving for independence but feels vulnerable. The child may have developed a number of social relationships based upon their early attachments. Children seem to form relationships with those people who are particularly responsive to their signals for attention and the child will initiate social exchanges with them. Research has shown that the amount of time that the adult spends with the child is not the important factor but it is the quality of the experience for the child during the period of adult contact which is most significant.

Signs of developmental delay at 18 months

Landers (1995) states that a doctor or health visitor should be consulted if the child shows any of the following signs of developmental delay at 18 months of age:

Fails to develop a mature heel-toe walking pattern after several months of walking
Does not speak at least 15 different words by 18 months
Does not use two-word sentences by age two
Does not seem to know the function of common household objects by 15 months
Does not imitate actions or words by the end of this period
Does not follow simple instructions by age two
Cannot push a wheeled toy by age two

(Landers, 1995)

18–24 Months

Physical development

The child's mobility in crawling, walking and running allows them independence as they move around the home. They will enjoy running ahead of their care-giver on the way to the park, where they will show off new abilities in scaling the climbing frame or balancing on small benches or slides. They will like to join in ball games with friends and siblings, although they will still not be physically co-ordinated enough to throw balls. There is increased eye–hand co-ordination and this is demonstrated in their added ability in reaching, grasping and manipulating objects by bringing them together and relating them to one another.

At 2 years the child has reached a stage whereby they can run safely, avoiding obstacles and stopping and starting easily. They are able to rise to their feet from a sitting position without using their hands. They like to express independence through climbing on to furniture to look through a window, or by opening cupboard doors and handling whatever comes to hand. When they walk upstairs and down they hold on to the rail or wall and put two feet on each step before moving forward. A small ball can be thrown but they will walk into a large ball when trying to kick it. Mealtimes also offer scope for more independence as they are able to lift and drink from a cup, replace it on the table and spoon feed themselves without spilling the food. The development of small muscle control is seen in the way the child removes wrappers, builds a tower of six or seven cubes, turns pages singly, scribbles spontaneously in circles and makes dots, imitates a vertical line and sometimes a letter V, puts on their hat and shoes and is able to turn door handles.

Intellectual development

Piaget would now describe the child as passing from the sensorimotor stage to the pre-operational stage and intuitive thinking. At 18 months they are aware of the practical relationships such as where objects are, where they were previously and where they belong. The child is able to indicate their nose, eyes, hair and shoes, and points to pictures of familiar objects such as a clock, a car or a dog. This transition from the sensorimotor to the pre-operational stage is characterized by symbolic games when the child imitates their own past actions in very simple, concrete ways which show that they have mental images of these actions, e.g. pretending to go to sleep, curling up their body and shutting their eyes. Their imagination develops as they learn to pretend to drink first from a cup, then another object unlike a cup. With a vocabulary of about 15 words and an understanding of many more they are able to show appreciation of speech by imitating certain words and trying to join in nursery rhymes. They can undress themselves and are able to use a word in order to vocalize their need to use the toilet.

They are able to put large square, round and triangular pegs into matching holes and can make shapes from clay. They are able to draw horizontal lines and make a 'train' by placing blocks horizontally. At age two they are able to use a chair as a means to an end, e.g. pushing it over to a shelf and standing on the chair to reach something on the shelf. Imitation is shown in the child's play when they copy the carer's domestic activities and they extend this symbolic play to their toys, which they pretend to put in bed to sleep. Piaget calls imaginative play 'the purest form of egocentric and symbolic thought'. Whilst it is egocentric in that the child is wrapped in their own dramatization, symbolic play leads them away from egocentricity because it enables them to feel what it is like to be something or someone else apart from themselves, e.g. a dog or an aeroplane. Egocentricity is a characteristic of the second major stage of intellectual development which Piaget calls the 'pre-operational thought period'.

Language development

At 2 years the child will have a vocabulary of about 50 words and can understand many more. They are able to put words together to make simple sentences, e.g. 'Daddy go car'. The child's curiosity seems insatiable as they continually ask the names of objects; the adult should answer questions in a meaningful way which can be understood by the child. Nursery rhymes, finger play, songs and pictures all help to stimulate the child's language.

Language development is dependent upon the child having a good learning environment and the interest of adults who will extend the child's language. Almost every part of the daily routine provides opportunities for extending children's vocabulary. The way adults speak to children and answer their questions will also have an effect upon the child's linguistic development. By about 30–36 months, children will have a vocabulary of over 200 words. Children will have struggled with the use of pronouns, recognizing themselves as 'I' being the most important, then 'he', 'she', 'it', 'you', 'we', 'they' and 'us'. Familiar objects may be identified in pictures and their function given, e.g. ball – throw, bounce. They will also repeat words that they may have heard in conversation but may not always understand the meaning of the words or where they should be used.

Emotional development

The child now experiences and exhibits a variety of emotions, pleasure, satisfaction, joy, anger, frustration, distress etc. as they struggle towards independence. They are still dependent upon adults for comfort and security, but the struggle between dependence and independence leads to temper tantrums. Temper tantrums are common between 18–36 months and need to be dealt with sensitively. The adult should not show anger during this phase as it is a developmental stage, but they can play a role in preventing tantrums. When dealing with children in a tantrum the adult should adopt a friendly tone of voice, request the child to do something rather than command them, and say 'please' and 'thank you' to the child. Adults should not over-react when the child says 'No', and should not offer the child choices when none exists. Wherever possible the child should be offered alternative distracting activities and if necessary be taken out of the room away from other children and adults. Adults should choose battles carefully and should avoid situations which could lead to a tantrum. Good behaviour should always be positively rewarded. After the tantrum is over the child should be hugged to make them feel secure and to let them know that the normal relationship has returned unchanged.

The child will show pleasure in possessions which they label as 'mine'. They gain pleasure from achievements such as looking at pictures and pointing to and naming objects they recognize such as dog, bus or car. They like the comfort of sitting on the adult's lap.

Social development

The child's social development depends upon the home and environmental influences of the child, for example, whether they have siblings, live in a house or high rise apartment, meet other children in the park or at the one-o-clock club, or have a large extended family with grandparents, cousins etc. nearby. At this stage everything revolves around the child's world and they cannot understand the concept of sharing with other children. The child is content to play alongside other children but not with them (parallel play).

Toilet training

Toilet training must be a gradual process and should never become a 'battleground' between adult and child. Habit formation via routine in early infancy should have laid a foundation for the regularity of meals, nappy changing, bath times and sleep times. At 15 months some children will indicate when they are wet and at 18 months they may be able to indicate beforehand. Before toilet training the child's physical development should be at a stage whereby they are able to sit comfortably on a potty and climb onto a chair. Negative reactions by carers on the child's lack of control can have an adverse effect on the child's learning abilities by giving them feelings of guilt or by the child trying too hard to please. It is helpful if the child is allowed to accompany a parent to the toilet in order to realize how natural it is. Bowel control is often achieved before bladder control as there are fewer bowel actions for the child to cope with. Some children may be dry at night by 2½–3 years; however, boys often take longer to achieve this than girls. Most children can keep dry during the day (with adult vigilance) by the age of 2½–3 years.

When an accident occurs it is best to mop it up without comment, the child should not be scolded. Instead the child should be praised when they warn you before the incident occurs, or even brings the potty to you. Patience and understanding are the prerequisite for the management of the 18-month-old child who is proceeding from the dependence of babyhood to the more independent toddler stage.

2½–3 Years

Physical development

At 2½ years of age the child can now run well and climb simple apparatus. They jump with their feet together, are able to stand on tiptoe and can kick a large ball. They can walk upstairs on their own but need to hold a rail when walking downstairs and still do this by putting two feet on each step. They are able to push and pull large wheeled toys but they are unable to steer them around obstacles. They have now developed fine muscle dexterity and can pick up pins and thread, build a tower of seven cubes and arrange blocks to form a train. They are able to hold a pencil or crayon and imitate drawing a horizontal line, letters T and V and a circle, and paint strokes, dots and circular

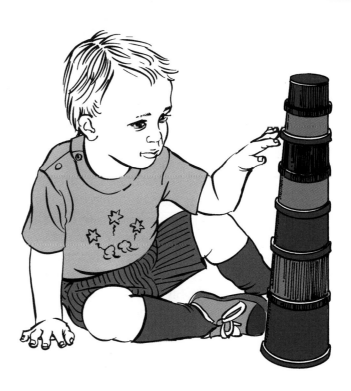

Building a tower of seven
pieces

shapes using an easel. At the table they are able to use a spoon skilfully
and may also be able to use a fork. They can pull their pants down to
go to the toilet but find it difficult to pull them up again. In their sand
and water play they enjoy filling jugs or other containers and tipping
the contents out again.

By 3 years the child can walk upstairs independently with alternating movements of the feet, although they will still come downstairs
two feet to a step and are able to jump from the bottom step. They are
able to climb apparatus at the nursery or swing park, can push and pull
large toys around corners and obstacles and can ride a tricycle and
steer it around wide corners. They can stand on one foot and sit cross-
legged. They are able to build small blocks into a tower of nine or
make deliberate patterns with them. They can scribble freely, imitate
circles, a cross, letters VHT, draw a man (usually a head and face with
projections for arms and legs), can cut with scissors and can confidently paint pictures using a large brush. They are able to eat with a
fork and spoon, and can carry their cup without spillage. They can
wash their hands but need help with drying them. They are able to
pull their pants up and down but need help to put on coats and
fastening zips and buttons. They like to play with clay and dough,
usually pounding and banging rather than making shapes.

Intellectual development

The child's increasing co-ordination of their body is important at this stage for the development of intelligence as the sensorimotor schemes concerned with body control form the base for intellectual development. For example, the ability to grasp one cube and place it on top of another leads to the development of concepts such as 'under', 'over', 'on top' and the way in which the movement of the lower object causes movement of the upper object which is resting upon it.

Those who believe in Piagetian-based child development theory will argue that children must be encouraged to explore and discover properties of play materials. Therefore activities such as threading beads, music and movement etc. develop the child's understanding of space and time as well as helping the development of their fine motor movements. Pre-reading and pre-number activities such as selection of clothes for dressing dolls and being able to put them on the doll in the right sequence, and setting the table with one plate and one mug for each child are more important to children at this age than teaching formal reading skills.

At 2½ years of age the child engages in domestic play such as putting toys to bed and washing clothes. They are very jealous of adult attention and whilst they may show interest in other children they do not have the notion of sharing playthings. Developing curiosity is seen in the frequency of questions beginning 'What?' and 'Where?'. The child has no concept of time and everything happens in the present.

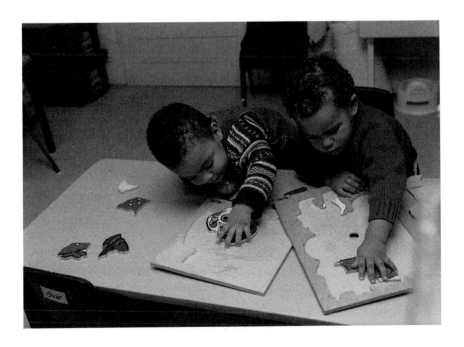

However, they are beginning to see themselves as a person and will ask 'Who?'. The child's motor ability enables them to build a tower of nine cubes, and after being shown a demonstration are able to build a 'train' with a chimney and a bridge (two blocks placed side by side with one placed in the middle on top of both). They are able to discriminate colours and can mix the primary colours (yellow, red and blue) to make new colours. They are able to match a circle, square and triangle on a form board.

They are able to carry out requests to do small tasks and get a sense of satisfaction when they have completed these. They begin to join in activities with other children but still prefer solitary and 'parallel' play. The child gradually comes to show an appreciation of past and present and they will describe experiences of 'last night', 'yesterday' etc. They like to pretend to tell the time by asking 'What time is it?', 'When is lunchtime?'.

At this stage the child is still marginally egocentric but as they progress further into the pre-operational phase new intellectual skills and knowledge enable the child to predict other people's thoughts and feelings. However, the child believes what they see, hear or experience at a given moment and are not able to apply what they have learnt in previous situations to the present.

During the first half of what Piaget calls the preconceptual thought stage the child is organizing their experiences into concepts such as time, space and number causality. In the second or intuitive phase they may be able to think in terms of grouping like objects together such as 'Apple, banana and orange are all fruit' but orange could also be put into the class of colour. The child will often use one word to describe a group of associated objects, for example calling all four legged animals dogs. Some children may refer to all men as 'daddy'.

Concepts of quantity use words such as 'more', 'less', 'all', 'some' or 'none', as at this stage they are unable to count in a meaningful way. Concepts of number are linked with the Piagetian stage of concrete operations and children who seem able to count from one to 10 are probably just enjoying the rhythmic jingle without having a concept of 'oneness' or 'threeness' etc.

Language development

By the age of 3 years the child is able to construct long sentences and can talk about situations in the past and in the future. They have a good command of vocabulary and this gives the child confidence. Some children may have infantile substitutions for certain letters (usually p, t, th, f, s, r, l, w, y) and the child may say, 'I will wun' or 'I will go for a wide' or 'Give me dat' or 'Put it dere'. The child should not be corrected at this age as it will inhibit their free flow of conversation. The child's language will now develop in relation to the total behaviour patterns of the child and the complexity or difficulty of the situations in which they find themselves and which they can deal with verbally. Starting at playgroup or nursery school will enhance their language development as they will learn new words alongside the new concepts.

Emotional development

This period is often described as 'the terrible twos' and/or the 'trusting threes'. At 2½ years the child is still swinging emotionally between positive and negative reactions. Sometimes they are rebellious, unco-operative and naughty and at other times they are dependent and clinging. Six months later they can be remarkably different, reacting in a co-operative, friendly and loving manner to adults and appearing to model themselves on adult behaviour. The 2½-year-old can be aggressive and may quarrel noisily with another child if they are both trying to use the same toy. At this age children do not always distinguish clearly between people and things, both of which they consider to be their possessions. They are interested in other children but may regard them like curiosities by poking, pushing, hugging and even licking them (tasting them)!

At around 2 years the child's imagination begins to develop. They may have dreams and nightmares and are unable to distinguish between fantasy and reality. When a child is 3 years their parents may have decided to have another child (a 3–4-year gap between children being the most popular in the UK). This may lead to the child experiencing sibling jealousy and rivalry. Jealousy arises when the child is frustrated by having to share the love of the parents and care-givers, whereas rivalry is the angry feeling which results when the child is frustrated in their desire to win. A new baby will make the youngest child jealous as they have been displaced from their position in the family and the feeling of rivalry may be felt towards an older sibling who is stronger and more able to cope, or the new arrival. Such feelings are quite natural and can be made less painful for the child if parents and care-givers are sensitive to the child's feelings. At any age a child should always be prepared in advance for the arrival of a new baby by parents and care-givers talking to the child, telling them stories, showing them pictures, pointing out other small babies and explaining to the child how dependent they are. Emphasis must be placed on the individuality of each child in the family and parents and care-givers should avoid competition or comparisons between children. It is also important to provide the child with the right play experiences so they can work out their feelings through play.

Social development

Between 2½–3 years is the time when most children will benefit socially by going to playgroup or nursery school. At this age they will usually attend for a morning or afternoon session. The mother or primary care-giver should always stay with the child when they first join the group as this will avoid the trauma of the first separation. Slowly the child will come to trust the staff in the nursery or playgroup, become interested in the toys and activities and will forget the presence of the mother or care-giver. It is at this point that the mother or care-giver can leave the child. It is important that the mother or care-giver is not late to collect the child at the end of the session; any lateness at this point will result in the child becoming distressed as they will feel lost and abandoned.

3–4 Years

Physical development

Large muscle control is seen in the child's ability to walk upstairs with alternating feet, march, run 10 steps with co-ordinated alternating arm movements, pedal a tricycle, somersault forward, kick a large ball when it is rolled to them, climb up and slide down a 1–2 m (4–6 feet) slide, jump from a height of 20 cm (8 inches), catch a ball with two hands and walk on tiptoe. The ability to use scissors has developed so

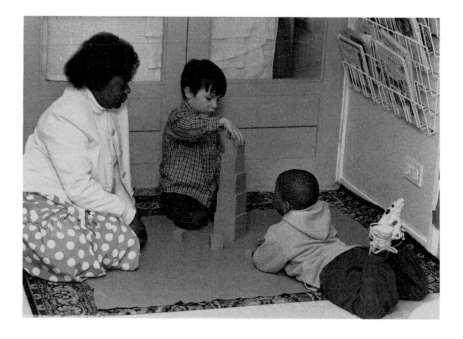

they are now able to cut along a 20 cm (8 inch) straight line within 1 cm (¼ inch) of the line. They are able to trace templates and put together a three-piece formboard or puzzle. The child has also developed further skills towards independence as they are able to use a knife, fork and spoon, brush their teeth, put on mittens, button and unbutton large buttons, put their coat on a hanger, and dress and undress themselves with some help with fasteners. All of the above indicate increasing development of the fine muscle movements and small muscle control.

Intellectual development

The child now has a large vocabulary, about 900 words and an understanding of many more. They will talk freely to themselves and others. Favourite words are 'Who?', 'What?', 'Where?' as they eagerly seek information about new aspects of their world such as the playgroup or nursery. The child's senses will add to their knowledge of the environment as they observe the actions of other children at play, and sometimes they will join in; they take part in music sessions and generally extend their play repertoire. The child's liking for imaginative play is seen in their keenness to dress up and role play in the home corner. The child's world of fantasy can be enhanced by stories, picture books, puppets, finger plays and songs. The child is now approaching Piaget's intuitive phase and beginning to form concepts as they play with sand, clay and water.

Scenario 6.1

Rory is a child-care student in a nursery school. Rory's tutor is paying a visit to the placement and asks Rory to describe the developmental value of outdoor play activities for 3–4-year-olds. Write an account of the answer that you would expect Rory to give to his tutor.

Time is first experienced in infancy as a series of events linked to the body rhythms and the patterns imposed by the environmental functions such as eating and sleeping. Later, actions which deal with a succession of objects, such as filling a cup with cubes at 18 months of age, or pushing and pulling a wheeled toy which starts and stops, all form the basis of time perception. Apart from the amount of time involved in these activities, the repetition of stimuli such as in music, dance or even rhythmically patting a baby in arms provide another kind of experience necessary for time concepts. An understanding of duration or an appreciation of the intervals in between events is also required for the development of a mature concept of time. Piaget states that the young child sees duration in terms of content rather than speed, which is the same idea we all share when it appears that pleasant events pass very quickly whilst painful or unhappy events seem to go on forever. At 3½ years the child can use past and future tenses correctly and is able to use complex expressions of duration such as 'for a long time', 'for a whole week'. The child can tell their carer that they go to playgroup 'on Fridays' and that they played 'only for a short time' in the sand pit, but they may still confuse yesterday and today: 'I'm going for a walk yesterday'. Tomorrow and future events are well understood by the 4-year-old child and they can recount recent events and experiences, although accounts are often a mixture of fact and fantasy.

It is important to note that children under 4 years of age cannot 'look forward' to events or even appreciate 'later this afternoon'. Adults often try to comfort a 3-year-old child on their first day in nursery school with expressions like, 'Don't worry I will come back soon' or 'Don't worry I will be back at 3 o'clock', when children have no concept of 'later' or '3 o'clock'. The child normally responds to these well-meant efforts by crying even louder as they see their carer disappear through the door in what to them is finality.

The child's concept of space is also derived from bodily experiences. In the sensorimotor stage the child looks, touches, grasps, feels, mouths and moves arms and legs, fingers and toes and trunk in order to gain concepts of their body and other objects. In the pre-operational stage their concept of space is egocentric, i.e. related to their body movements and perceptions. The distance between the child and an object will influence the child's judgement of the object's size and their own size. The child tends to judge a close object as larger than it actually is and distant objects as smaller. Playing with blocks, trucks, tricycles and mobile toys helps the child to perceive short distances accurately, but they cannot judge long distances unrelated to their own body size. Concepts of relative size enable children between the ages of 3 and 4 years to select the biggest and the smallest of a small selection of items.

Children's use of spatial terms is also linked with vertical orientation, for example, when they are shown toy models of a dog and a horse they have no doubts that the horse is the biggest, however, if the dog is placed on a box making it higher than the horse they will say that the dog is the biggest provided that they have seen the dog being moved. However, if at the start they are shown the animals with the horse on the ground and the dog on the box they will get the right answer by saying that the horse is the biggest. It would appear that moving the dog upwards whilst the child watches makes the child think 'vertically' and therefore 'big' means tall or high. Another explanation of this experiment is the child does not understand the different concepts which are expressed by the words 'big' and 'high' or 'big' and 'tall' and therefore uses the wrong descriptor.

The concept of causality refers to the child's ability to explain events of the outside world. At the egocentric stage the child explains everything in personal terms as they perceive them. Sometimes the child will involve people close to them or, if they have been told about God, they will quote God as the cause of a number of events, so a 4-year-old child trying to explain 'night' says that 'God has put the lights out'. Of course much of this type of thinking stems from the explanations that adults have given to the child in answer to those 'Where?', 'How?', 'Why?' questions. A more accurate answer of the reason for night from a child that has had their questions answered in an honest fashion may be 'The sun has gone to bed'.

Language development

By 4 years of age the child has a vocabulary of some 1500–2000 words, talks in sentences and continually asks questions. Language development during this period is rapid and the child talks, plays with words, comments; makes simple responses into long narratives, criticizes, balances comparisons etc. All situations are likely to be verbalized, even block play and drawing. The child's language is now moving beyond their egocentrism and their immediate situation. The child is able to blend sounds together, an ability which is important for learning to read. The child uses complete sentences, e.g. 'The tree is outside', 'The grass is wet'. The adult can learn a great deal by listening to the child's conversations with other children. If the child is unable to communicate successfully with their peers then their self-confidence is likely to suffer.

Emotional development

At 3 years of age the child emerges from their identity conflicts as a trusting, generally friendly person who will now join in play with other children, show affection for younger siblings and be willing to share some of their toys. They like to help around the house and garden and reveal their feelings through imaginative play. As the child's self-confidence increases at 4 years they may show reluctance to follow the wishes of an adult and give cheeky answers when reproved. Although they prefer to play with other children they are also capable of being aggressive towards them. The child does learn to share and knows that they cannot be first all the time and has to take turns with other children and share the attention of the adult. The child is able to show compassion for other children by comforting a crying baby or a newcomer to the nursery. This compassion develops further as they get older. By 4 years the child will not only be confident but may be the senior in the playgroup, and in this position may show a friendly kindly interest in the younger children and enjoy being praised by adults for being 'sensible'. The child will model their behaviour on the adults around them, therefore if the adults present a confusing, inconsistent environment the child will find it difficult to trust them. Even though they may be the 'senior' the child will still turn to adults for comfort when they are tired, hurt, afraid or ill.

Social development

The age of 3 years has traditionally been regarded as the ideal age for a child to enter a play group or nursery school, as by this time the child is ready to extend their social relationships. However, as mentioned earlier, some children may reach this stage at 2½ years and others at 5 years.

At the 4-year-old stage, children tend to play in groups, but the focus of interest is the activity rather than the other children. These are not permanent groups; children will play together in a particular project, i.e. constructing a spaceship, then they will drift to another group for another activity. Four-year-olds like to tell long stories, often about everyday events, but most of which is pure imagination. Some adults become annoyed when, having believed a story as the truth and maybe having taken action as a result of the events they have heard about, have found out later from the child that it was pure fantasy. On the other hand some parents/carers will worry about the child telling lies when they are indulging in their fantasy stories. A lively imagination is of great benefit to the child as it enables them to solve problems of loneliness, jealousy and other matters that may be bothering them. Children will often invent an imaginary friend or companion; this may be in the form of a pet, adult or other child. Parents/carers and siblings are expected to accept the newcomer to the family and it will be the newcomer who will be blamed for naughty deeds and often used to draw attention to the child who may be feeling neglected. Alternatively the imaginary playmate may express the child's wishes to be grown up and powerful or naughty and babyish. Most parents/carers allow the child to outgrow the imaginary playmate, but if the playmate becomes too obstructive it may be necessary to set limits upon what it is allowed to do.

The socialization process by which a child accepts the customs, manners and traditions of the family, culture and peer group, enabling them to be accepted as a member of society, involves two aspects that are sometimes seen as controversial: gender stereotyping and the idea that boys and girls are expected to behave differently. A lot has been written about both these areas and specific references can be found at the end of this chapter. Both parents and carers should give the same opportunities for play to boys and girls. Girls need the skills of learning to ride a bicycle and climbing as much as boys need the skills of cooking and learning to push a pram. Children choose toys from interest not because they are 'boys'' toys or 'girls'' toys. It is the influence of adults around them that will lead children to view certain toys as unacceptable. Small boys enjoy playing with dolls, but it is the negative reactions of their parents/carers which will lead them to believe that they should not play with dolls.

Scenario 6.2

Maria is a nursery nurse in a nursery school. Eamon aged 4¼ years has thrown the Lego all over the floor and is refusing to pick it up. Eamon says that he did not do it but Curly did it. There is no child in the nursery called Curly.

Write an explanation of what you think is happening here and how Maria should deal with Eamon.

4–5 Years

Physical development

At this stage the child develops and extends their existing skills. They are able to stand on one foot without aid for 4–8 seconds, are able to walk a balance beam, hop on one foot five successive times, jump backwards six times and jump forward 10 times without falling. Large muscle control is demonstrated when the child is able to run, change direction, jump over a string 5 cm (2 inches) from the floor, bounce and catch a large ball, walk downstairs with alternating feet and pedal a tricycle, which they can steer around corners. Manual dexterity is seen in their ability to make clay shapes which are put together in two or three parts, cut along a curved line, cut out a 5 cm (2 inch) circle, cut out and paste simple shapes and draw simple recognizable pictures such as a house, man or tree. The child can wash and dry their hands and face, dress and undress alone, count the fingers on one hand using the index finger of the other hand, use correct utensils for eating food, carry out toilet activities unaided, put on and sometimes do up shoes (although for many children tying laces will be a skill which they only become adept at much later) and help set the table for meals.

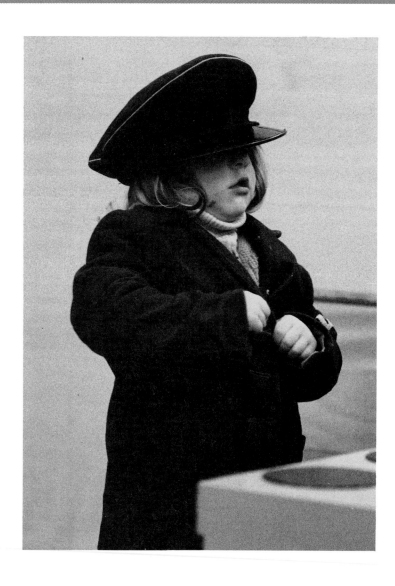

Dressing up activities provide opportunities for developing manual dexterity (4–5 years).

Intellectual development

Between the age of 4–5 years, after demonstration, children can build a tower of 10 blocks and any number of three-block bridges when requested. Building vertically is easier at this stage than making horizontal rows. It has been suggested that this may be due to the vertical space orientation of the body which remains constant in an up-and-down sense, whereas the environment of left and right sides changes constantly.

At age 5 years, children transfer from the nursery school or class into the infants school. This moving on should be a natural sequence and should not cause the child distress. The child should have previously visited the school and met with the head and class teacher. If a child has not attended nursery school or playgroup then they are likely

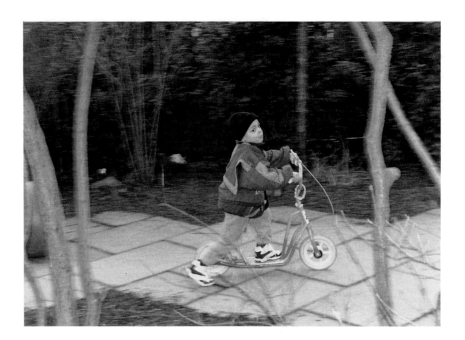

to find the transition to school a difficult and distressful event. As approximately 80% of all 4-year-olds are attending school either full time or on a sessional basis, it would be very rare to find a 5-year-old child who had no pre-school/school experiences. More details regarding the effects of school on children's intellectual development can be found in Chapter 7. They are able to join in group activities and like games which have rules (although they may choose to disregard these if they are not winning!). At this age children often become bored with nursery activities and will need to be stretched intellectually to overcome this.

Language development

The child may have a vocabulary of around 3000 words, and asks many questions. They like to demonstrate their oral abilities and often test adults' reactions to 'bad language'. Parents/carers usually react with horror when a child uses a swear word and always insist that they did not hear it at home or nursery. Children are able to pick up swear words from radio, TV, listening to adults in shops and other children. Parents/carers should not punish children for swearing; in the first instance they should ignore the child, but if it persists the child does need to be told that it is unacceptable language for the nursery or home. The child is able to classify in a more sophisticated manner, knowing the makes of cars, or names of flowers and trees, depending on where there special interest lies. Many children are interested in dinosaurs and it is interesting how they remember and correctly pronounce the very complicated names of the different types of dinosaurs.

Emotional development

At this age the child is kind and protective towards younger children and pets. They enjoy stories that have strong and powerful people and they also like stories which have monsters and ghosts and may be scary but thrilling for them. They develop friendships with other children and want to be part of a group. They are beginning to understand that not all adults react in the same way and that adults have feelings too.

Social development

Between 4–5 years of age the child may change from a stable, friendly nursery 'senior' into a noisy, rude, boastful extrovert. This is often a defensive reaction to the major changes that they are undergoing as they enter school and find that the children there are so much bigger than them. Peer groups now become very important and they are often motivated in their behaviour by peer group pressure and the need to have the approval of the peer group. Group games often become competitive, and the adult may need to act as the referee. They begin to understand cultural differences and that not all families are the same.

Scenario 6.3

Naghina is a student child care worker in a nursery school. The teacher has asked her to devise a project for a group of 4¼–5-year-olds.
  What developmental stages should Naghina take into account when devising the project?

When they reach primary school stage not all children have reached the same stage of development. There can be a wide variety of development stages in children of this age group depending upon their previous experience, environment and ability. Some children may appear to be ahead of others by being able to read, but it may also be found that these children may not be ahead in everything, for example they may be behind in manual skills and need help with dressing. For children in this position it can be very distressing to find that there are things they are unable to do; careful and sensitive handling is necessary as they will need a lot of encouragement. Most children have motor skills and control of their large muscles which enable them to walk a balance board forwards, backwards and sideways, skip, swing on a swing initiating and sustaining motion, climb stepladders or steps to a slide, dribble a ball, kick a football, ride a bicycle, slide on a sledge, jump a rope, steer a wagon propelling it with one foot, walk or play in waist-high water in the swimming pool, jump up and pivot on one foot, jump from a height of 12 inches and land on the balls of their feet, stand on one foot without support and eyes closed and hang from a horizontal bar bearing their weight on their arms.

Small muscle control enables most children to spread their fingers, touch their thumb to each finger, copy small letters, print large capital letters anywhere on the paper, hit a nail with a hammer, colour in an outline staying within the lines for 95% of the picture, cut pictures from magazines or catalogue without being more than ¼ inch from the edge, use a pencil sharpener, copy complex drawings, tear simple shapes from paper, fold a paper square twice on the diagonal in imitation, catch a soft ball or bean bag with one hand, hit a ball with a bat or stick, print their name on lined paper, open a carton of milk, buckle their own car seat belt and serve themselves and others with breakfast cereal.

Intellectual development

Starting school should promote the intellectual needs of 5-year-olds. At school they will learn to adapt skills which they practised at home or nursery such as eating, drinking, dressing, undressing, going to the toilet and washing their hands. Intellectual growth progresses with the maturation of the central nervous system. The 5–6-year-old age group marks a period of rapid physical and intellectual growth. The maturation process needs to be reached before a child can reach a developmental stage, and factors such as diet, poverty, wealth and environment may all have an effect upon the rate of maturation. Education is a stimulus for the growth of intelligence; however, other factors also play a role such as genetics, experiences of the child etc. It is necessary for child care workers to recognize the differences in children's ability and accept that there is no educational process which can bring all children up to the same level. The effective child care worker, parent or teacher appreciates the differing ages, stages, interests and needs of each child in order that they can benefit as much as possible from their education.

As egocentrism decreases so the child begins to see causes as impersonal and their understanding progresses from the concrete to a more abstract thought. This is the stage which Piaget referred to as the intuitive phase. At this stage children will explain events by a description or offer a number of different causes for an event, as they may have difficulty in understanding the concept of impersonal cause. Piaget described the tendency of children to attribute living qualities to inanimate objects as 'animistic thinking'. Adults often encourage children in this and television also encourages animistic thinking as the children see stories of animated toys, trains and animals.

Piaget wrote about the child's stages of development in relation to the principles of conservation. Adults accept that the amount of a substance remains unchanged even when its shape is changed or when it is divided into parts. Children from 4–7 years do not have this concept. The child's conservation of mass can be demonstrated by giving a child some clay and asking them to make a ball the same size as an existing ball that they can see as a model. When the child is asked whether the two balls are of the same size they will reply 'yes'. One ball is then rolled into a long sausage shape and the child will now state that the sausage shape contains more clay than the other ball because it is longer (therefore 'bigger' or 'more').

Language development

Children now have a large vocabulary which serves to unify the different aspects of their behaviour. They are able to count up to 10, know the names of the more familiar colours, give their name, age, birthday and home address when asked. They are also developing other skills relating to language such as listening, speaking, reading and writing. The child will learn and use new words learnt at school and will also gain new words from books, poetry, stories and television.

Emotional development

Starting school may prove exciting and/or scary for children depending on their previous experiences away from home. Although the school may use informal learning methods there will be a lot of formal learning taking place alongside the informal. Children take a while to settle down, but once they have developed a trust and formed secure relationships with the teacher and the other staff they will regain their self-confidence. For many children the teacher becomes an important part of their lives, and many parents and carers will hear the teacher's thoughts on every subject from wellingtons to gerbils as quoted by the child.

Social development

Children who have had experience at nursery or playgroup will be used to making new friends and being away from their parents for part of the day. However, in spite of all the right pre-school experiences some children do not adapt to school. School can offer the excitement of new equipment and activities, but the child will get less attention from adults compared with the nursery. Teachers have considerable responsibilities to develop children's skills and teach them new knowledge and skills; carrying this out efficiently leaves very little time to spend on a one-to-one basis with individual children. Some children may miss this individual attention and this may lead them to behaving in a way which attracts the attention of the teacher. As the term proceeds so the child will make friends and will introduce these friends to their parents or carers; the child may be invited to other friends' homes for tea or birthday parties. At this stage children are aware of the differences in adults and home life and are beginning to understand that they have to behave in a manner which is acceptable to a large number of adults.

Scenario 6.4

Melanie has been learning in college about Piaget's theories relating to the child's development of the concept of conservation of mass.

Devise an experiment that Melanie can use in her placement to illustrate Piaget's theory.

6–7 Years

Physical development

At 6 years of age the average height of the child is 1.07 m and their weight is 18.14 kg. This is a period of rapid growth and 'filling out'; a similar process happens in adolescence. The development of motor skills during this stage depends less upon informal, spontaneous learning and more upon the learning of rules for formalized activities. There is now a change in the classroom setting and children have to sit longer and concentrate more on what they are learning. The child's muscle co-ordination and balance continues to improve as physical exercise is enjoyed for its own sake rather than as a competition with peers. Team games, e.g. football, rounders, skipping and hopscotch are popular, and both boys and girls should be encouraged to play all of these.

Intellectual development

The concept of conservation of weight and volume is more difficult than that of mass and most children cannot grasp this until they are 6 years of age or older. Children around the ages of 6–7 years can usually accurately answer the questions related to conservation shown in Table 6.4.

Table 6.4 Conservation tests

1 Conservation of substance	
A	**B**
The adult presents two identical clay balls. The child agrees that they are equal amounts of clay.	One of the balls is rolled out to form another shape. The child is asked whether they still contain equal amounts.
2 Conservation of length	
A	**B**
Two sticks are aligned in front of the child. The child agrees they are equal.	One of the sticks is moved to the right. The child is asked whether they are still the same.
——————— ———————	——————— ———————
3 Conservation of number	
A	**B**
Two rows of counters are placed in one-to-one correspondence. The child admits they are equal.	One of the rows is spread out or brought closer together. The child is asked whether each row still has the same number.

They are now not only able to recognize different shapes but know the properties of these shapes.

Language development

At this age they are able to recall part of a story, speak in sentences with more than five words, use the future tense, tell longer stories. They will speak up for themselves at the doctor or dentist and will enjoy making decisions. They have new words relating to mathematical and scientific concepts and are able to discuss these with adults. They enjoy conversations with their friends and like adults have an enjoyment for 'gossip' such as who has which new toy and where other children have been on outings or which TV programme they may have watched.

Emotional development

At 6 years of age the child can appear less stable than they were at 5 years of age. The child may be irritable, self-centred and aggressively refuse to share toys and books. At times they may rebel against rules and the limits on behaviour set by teachers or parents. The child loves to tackle new skills like computer techniques but they may become frustrated if they find them difficult.

Social development

This is the stage of Erikson's 'industry' versus 'inferiority' which lasts from 6-9 years, when the child's circle of significant relationships revolves around the school and the neighbourhood. During this phase the child discovers not only that they are a distinct person but that they are able to do things by themselves or with others. The child will take every opportunity to learn to become 'someone' in their imagination such as a pop star, doctor, fire fighter, astronaut or police officer. They become very keen on the world around them and in gaining approval from adults.

Signs of developmental delay at 6 years

Landers (1995), whilst pointing out that each child develops in an individual manner, suggests that if a 6-year-old displays any of the following signs of possible developmental delay than a doctor or health visitor should be consulted:

Exhibits extremely fearful or timid behaviour
Exhibits extremely aggressive behaviour
Is unable to separate from parents without major protest
Is easily distracted and unable to concentrate on any single activity for more than five minutes
Shows little interest in playing with other children
Refuses to respond to people in general or responds only superficially
Rarely uses fantasy or imitation in play
Seems unhappy or sad much of the time
Does not engage in a variety of activities
Avoids or seems aloof with other children and adults
Does not express a wide range of emotions
Has trouble eating, sleeping or using the toilet
Seems unusually passive
Cannot understand two-part commands
Cannot correctly give her first and last names
Does not use plurals or past verb tense properly when speaking
Does not talk about her daily activities and experiences
Cannot build a tower of six to eight blocks
Seems uncomfortable holding a pencil

(Landers, 1995)

7–8 Years

Physical development

Physical growth continues but not as rapidly as in the earlier stages. Physical skills increase through informal play and more formal games with rules and teamwork. This is a time when co-operation rather than competition should be encouraged in games. Very physical play such as that in adventure playgrounds should also be provided as this is an outlet for frustration and aggression.

Intellectual development

The stage from 7–11 years is Piaget's period of 'concrete operations' when the acquisition of concepts shows progression from the pre-operational thought period. The child is now able to classify (group objects or events with similar properties) and from this understand the meaning of numbers and symbols. However, they will not be able to think of numbers hypothetically; they will still need concrete things to count. Concepts of colour are grasped more easily than concepts of form or shape. Learning to read and write demands attention to form and shape. The child has now reached a stage in development when they are able to sort by form or shape and then by colour; this also means that by the time they are eight they are able to perceive form, colour and size in an abstract way. Concepts of direction are still difficult for children under 8 years. When they are asked where their home or school is they may be able to give the address, but actual directions may only be 'over there' or 'near the bus stop'. Children need to do a lot of work using real directional situations to help them to develop directional ability. Children only really understand the concept of right and left between the ages of 7–8 years.

Emotional development

The child is now becoming increasingly confident as they become adept at new skills such as reading, writing, tying knots and bows, climbing trees, swinging on ropes and balancing on the equipment in adventure playgrounds. They like stories about the wonders and myths of magic, wizards, heroes and heroines and fables. They enjoy dramatic interpretation and may need restraining from too literal a translation of their particular idol's pursuits! This stage of development is a time of great joy and enthusiasm for life and the discovery of nature and the world around them. At this stage children begin to become aware of morality, i.e. knowing the difference between right and wrong.

Social development

Both girls and boys adopt heroes and can reel off the names of current pop stars, football stars, TV personalities etc. Children of this age like to write and receive letters; this may need some encouragement at first but they get a great pleasure from receiving their own letters through the mail box. Children also know that letters are a good way of conveying thoughts and feelings to others and thus being able to share pleasures. Some children may appear to be natural leaders and this should be discouraged as it is important that leadership is shared. The school should offer a climate of co-operation rather than competition.

| Assignments | 1. Choose two well known child development theorists and give a brief résumé of their theories. |

1. Choose two well known child development theorists and give a brief résumé of their theories.

2. Undertake five observations of a 3-month-old baby. Compare your results with the information on development in this chapter and Chapter 5. From the comparison write an evaluation of the observations.

3. What might be the signs of developmental delay in a child aged 18 months?

4. Why are the expressions 'terrible twos' and 'trusting threes' used to describe children aged 2 years and 3 years?

5. Describe the language development of a 4-year-old.

6. What does Piaget's stage of 'concrete operations' mean?

7. How should the parent/carer deal with the child's transition from playgroup to school so that it is as smooth and untraumatic as possible?

8. Write an essay on why it is important for children to learn to be co-operative rather than competitive.

REFERENCES AND FURTHER READING

Bee, Helen (1992). *The Developing Child*, 6th edition. Harper Collins, New York.

Browne, Naima and France, Pauline (1986). *Untying the Apron Strings: anti-sexist provision for the under fives*. Open University Press, Milton Keynes.

Dunn, Judy and Kendrick, Carol (1982). *Siblings: love envy and understanding*. Grant MacIntyre, London.

Faragher, Joan and MacNaughton, Glenda (1990). *Working with Young Children: guidelines for good practice*. TAFE Publications, Victoria, Australia.

Fatchett, Anita (1995). *Childhood to Adolescence: caring for health*. Baillière Tindall, London.

Grabrucker, Marianne (1988). *There's a Good Girl: gender stereotyping in the first three years of life: a diary*. The Women's Press, London.

Gross, Richard D. (1992). *Psychology: the science of mind and behaviour*. Hodder and Stoughton, London.

Landers, Cassie (1995). Childhood trainers: guide to the development of the young child. In *Enhancing the Skills of Early Trainers Pack*. Bernard van Leer Foundation/UNESCO Holland.

Leach, Penelope (1988). *Baby and Child: from birth to age 5 years*. Penguin, London.

Lindon, Jennie (1993). *Child Development from Birth to Eight: a practical focus*. National Children's Bureau, London.

Martorano, S.C. (1977). A developmental analysis of performance as Piaget's formal operations tasks. *Developmental Psychology* **13**, 666–672.

Phillips, Angela (1993). *The Trouble with Boys: parenting the men of the future*. Pandora, London.

Reid, Joanna (1995). More than meets the eye. New research into babies. *Nursery World*, 23 November, p. 12.

Williams, Kate and Gardner, Ruth (1994). *Caring for Children*. Pitman Publishing, London.

Chapter 7

Children's Play and Education

This chapter covers underpinning knowledge for parts of the following units for the National Vocational Qualifications (NVQs) in Child Care and Education: C8, C9, E1, P2, M7.
This chapter is also linked to CACHE awards modules: Diploma Modules: B, H, S; Certificate Modules: 2, 7, 8, 10

INTRODUCTION

Friedrich Froebel (1782–1852) was probably one of the first people to recognize that children's play was more than just something that the child did in order to pass the time but that it was actually a serious and deeply significant activity for young children. Susan Isaacs (1885–1948) wrote:

> If we were asked to mention one supreme psychological need of the young child, the answer would have to be 'play' – the opportunity for free play in all its various forms. Play is the child's means of living and of understanding life.
>
> (Isaacs, 1954)

In 1987, John Brierley, through careful study of the development of children's brains stated:

> All forms of play appear to be essential for the intellectual, imaginative and emotional development of the child and may well be necessary steps to a further stage of development.
>
> (Brierley, 1987)

A further acknowledgement of the importance of play is reflected in the United Nations Convention on the Rights of the Child, Article 31, which states:

> Every child is entitled to rest and play and to have the chance to join in a wide range of activities.
>
> (Department of Health, 1993)

From the above quotes and the significant contributions made by their authors to the field of child development there can be no doubt of the effects of play upon the child's psychological, intellectual, linguistic, emotional and social development.

As play is a powerful medium for learning it is important that all child care workers understand the value to the child of different types of play and how to present play activities that are appropriate to a child's stage of development. Through play children learn skills, gain concepts and understanding and draw relationships between concepts. They are able to practise problem solving and decision making, and learn how to successfully interact with other children and adults. They are able to build up their vocabulary and learn to express their ideas in words. There are four essential provisions needed for a child to have good play and learning experiences:

◆ A range of rich experiences
◆ An environment with interesting material and equipment relevant to the age and stage of development of the child
◆ An atmosphere in which each child is allowed to proceed at their own pace
◆ Understanding adults who are able to facilitate meaningful play experiences for the child

ROLE OF THE ADULT IN PLAY

The adult has an important role in providing an interesting, safe and suitable play environment for the child. There should be adequate space for the child to be able to manipulate equipment. Whilst the adult will structure some of the play activities there also needs to be other materials that are easily accessible for the child to introduce into the activity. For example, the adult may have set up the water-play area with the appropriate equipment to enable the child to strain, float, sink, pour, turn waterwheels etc. However, the child may decide to introduce some bricks in order to build a dam or use the water to wash the dolls and this will only be possible if the child has easy access to the bricks and dolls. If children do not come up with their own ideas for extending the play activity then the adult may offer suggestions. In this instance the adult's role is that of a facilitator who is able to provide an activity, observe and listen to the way the children use the activity and if necessary offer some new ideas in order to make the activity more challenging for the children.

Adults do need to intervene in children's play when it becomes dangerous or too boisterous, and in this case the role of the adult is to set boundaries/limits upon the children's actions or behaviour. The adult has a role in listening carefully to the children's use of language whilst they are playing and offering new words/descriptions.

Athey (1990) maintains that if adults observe children they will notice that the child exhibits 'a pattern of repeatable behaviour into which experiences are assimilated' and she calls these 'schema'. Athey identifies seven types of schema:

◆ Dynamic circular
◆ Dynamic vertical
◆ Dynamic back and forth, side to side
◆ Going over and under
◆ Going round a boundary
◆ Enveloping and containing
◆ Going through a boundary

The role of the adult is to recognize the schema and provide activities for the child that will enable them to pursue their particular schema. For example, if a child is working on a schema of enveloping and containing they will need activities which will enable them to extend the schema such as empty boxes, digging in the garden, wrapping parcels, putting dolls to bed etc.

A great deal of nursery practice requires the adult to be 'non-directive' and the activities to be 'child directed'. This usually means that the adult's role is to provide a stimulating environment and interesting materials and equipment to which the child will respond if they wish. This view overlooks the very important role that the adult can play if they become involved in children's play. Materials should be made available in such a way that the child's curiosity leads them to explore, discover various properties of the play equipment and ask questions about their findings. The adult helps the children clarify concepts and corrects misconceptions. Provision for individual differences in the child's learning style and rate are made as the adult helps the child towards problem solving in a way that corresponds to the child's developmental stage.

It is often difficult to determine the difference between a positive form of intervention and the adult interfering in the child's play. If comments are made too often, children become dependent upon the adult and stop playing when the adult moves to another group. If there is too much adult interference the children will lose interest and ownership in the play.

Adults' questions to children should be open ended (i.e. not allow a 'yes' or 'no' or one syllable answer) in order to extend the children's language and thinking. Examples of open ended questions could be:

♦ 'What are you going to do with this?' (stating the problem)
♦ 'How will you manage to put all those bricks into the wheel-barrow?' (testing understanding)
♦ 'Why did you have two wheelbarrows yesterday?' (recall)
♦ 'What do you think will happen if you pile them all in the small wheelbarrow?' (prediction)
♦ 'Why did we need two wheelbarrows yesterday?' (recap process)
♦ 'Which way is easiest for workers to move all these bricks?' (imaginative)

Any comments made by the adults should extend the child's learning, encourage thinking and clarify concepts.

When the adult answers children's questions they must be honest in their answers. If the adult does not know the answer to a child's question then they should tell the child that they do not know and suggest that they set up an experiment to find out or go together to the library to look up the answer. This does mean that child care workers need to understand the concepts themselves, such as why different objects sink and float, why plants cannot grow without light, what happens to the hamster when it dies, and how aeroplanes fly. Due to the influence of media such as television many more children are very knowledgeable about a great number of things and this can lead to children asking very sophisticated questions for which they want answers.

Imaginative play offers a lot of scope for adult involvement if they are invited by the children to join in the game. Children often invite adults into the home corner for tea or to buy goods at the classroom shop. Involvement in imaginative play enables the adult to extend the children's verbal skills and add an extra dimension to the imaginative process.

Repetition of routine activities will provide a sense of security for young children, but the timetable must be flexible to enable children to finish a project or go on outings or enjoy spontaneous play.

The adult has a role in the organization and supervision of children's play. Staff should work as a team and plan activities at least 1 week ahead. Many nursery schools and classes will have long-term activities such as outings, concerts and sports days, which have to be slotted into the timetable throughout the year and may not fit with the learning theme for a particular term.

Scenario 7.1

You are a nursery nurse in a local nursery school working with a group of 4-year-olds. Part of your role is to work with the teacher in planning activities for the children. Activities are usually based upon a theme; the theme for this term is Winter. The teacher has asked you to draw up a list of activities for 1 week based upon this theme and to state the likely learning outcomes for the children.

Activities are usually organized on a monthly or weekly basis and are planned to fit in with the learning theme. With the emphasis now being on the early years, curriculum activities are often accompanied by the learning outcomes/goals for the children. Some early years establishments with 4-year-olds are likely to be working towards the national desirable learning outcomes for children's learning on entering compulsory schooling which are assessed when the child reaches infants school. (Further reference to these is made later in the chapter.)

When planning learning outcomes these should be achievable by the majority of children. Special needs children in the nursery may need extra help in order to achieve specific outcomes. Examples of learning outcomes are as follows:

◆ Recognizing the motif on their own coat peg
◆ Counting to five and having an understanding of fiveness
◆ Identifying the colours blue, red and green

Activities will be chosen that will give the children the knowledge and skills needed to achieve the outcomes. For example, in learning to count to five and understand fiveness they will learn rhymes, songs, stories that involve numbers and counting, activities using five bricks, playing in groups of five children, cooking five cakes, learning the names of five days of the week etc.

Careful observation of a child's activities enables the adult to approach the child at the right level and enables the child to utilize their experiences with various materials. The adult can encourage the child to discuss their work, although adults must be careful not to make negative remarks about a child's work as this will damage the child's self-confidence.

Adults also have a role to ensure that the play environment is safe, removing broken toys, leaking water trays etc.

DEVELOPMENT THROUGH PLAY

As already stated, play is the child's main medium for learning and as such has implications for all aspects of development. All activities that the child undertakes are learning situations, therefore adults should never say, 'We'll finish this first and then you can play' as this draws an unnatural divide which suggests that some activities are more important than others, e.g. reading books is learning whereas dressing up is play.

Physical Development

The child benefits from play as it helps them to acquire body control. Co-ordination develops through movement and exercise. Random movements become purposeful as the child grasps a moving object. Later they progress from crawling to walking and running, from standing on one foot to hopping, and eventually to more complicated games requiring physical skills with large and small muscle movements.

Intellectual Development

The child is able to develop new skills and abilities with words and objects, experiment with the properties of creative media and play equipment and solve problems in their own way. Exploratory play begins at the breast with the most primitive senses of touch and taste, then proceeds through random movements to voluntary control of the hands, arms and legs which enables the child to grasp, hold and

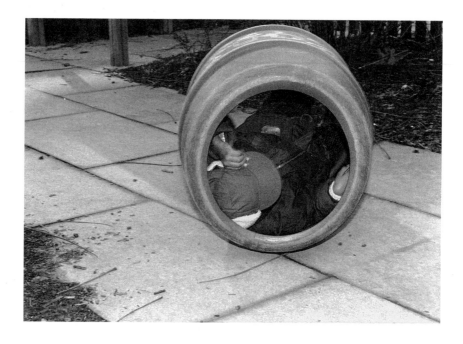

examine small objects. Through these movements the baby comes to acquire control over their body and attempts to control the environment as they progress from crawling to walking and running. They discover textures of food and other materials first by putting them in their mouth, later by feeling and close examination. Different shapes and sizes come to recognition as they try to grasp the coloured mobiles strung above their cot. Experimentation begins as they pull the cord which will set the chime bar into action and introduce another dimension, sound, into the activity.

Play with sound develops with the child's own babbling which is obviously a pleasurable activity apart from its later significance as a means of communication. Concepts of colour, form, size and properties of different play materials leads them to classify and categorize items to their own criteria. Eagerly they question in their enthusiasm to learn. A discovery, such as the necessity to add water to sand before one can build with it, is as important to the child as any discovery made by Archimedes. Emotional aspects are closely interwoven in their pride at achievement, and the adult should express the appropriate appreciation of their efforts.

Emotional Development

Play provides an outlet for feelings and the child can use playthings on which to vent their anger; smacking teddy, kicking the ball or pounding clay is preferable to the child punching other children or adults, or breaking plates and ornaments. As they develop they learn to use anger in a constructive way, hammering nails into wood or making clay models.

Play involves not only the negative feelings of fear, aggression, anxiety, hate, guilt and frustration, but also pleasure, happiness, exuberance, love and affection. Sometimes children have ambivalent feelings towards their parents; 'I don't love you anymore' or 'I hate you' are often said by children as they enter a power struggle which may revolve around a simple matter such as parents not allowing them a second slice of cake. Sometimes children will turn towards quiet peaceful activities such as jigsaw puzzles, stacking toys, Lego, water play or the book corner. This ability to use objects for their own needs will enable the child to cope with difficulties in future life.

Language Development

Play is a very powerful tool for the development of children's language. Bee (1992) points out that a number of researchers have noted the relationships between the patterns of children's play and their language development. Through play children develop new concepts, and with each concept there is a set of associated descriptive words.

Young children may often have a gap between the number of concepts which they have and the number of words at their disposal in order to describe these concepts. In other words, children often have an understanding of more concepts than they are able to describe. As children learn new words they incorporate these into their play and the play becomes more complex. Children often understand many more words than they are able to speak. Children may use language in their play in order to develop social relationships with other children and with adults. Through play children are able to practice their language ability and particular types of play, for example doll play, home corner, co-operative play, imaginative play, and these offer opportunities for the child to try out new words and sentences. Adults have an important role in extending children's language through play activities and introducing new words. Through play children are able to learn the language of problem solving, with the adult answering questions and offering simple explanations for the 'how', 'why', 'what' questions. As they get older (4–5 years old) children will use language in play situations to ask complicated questions, negotiate with other children, to explain what they are doing or what they intend to do next, to express their thoughts aloud, and to give instructions to others. Between the ages of 6–8 years they will use language to introduce rules into their games and ensure that all players keep to the rules.

Social Development

The process of socialization develops throughout the child's life. In the first years of life, children learn to socialize with the immediate members of their own family; when they go to playgroup or nursery, they then learn to socialize with other children and adults outside the family circle. Many children soon discover in this situation that what has been acceptable behaviour within their own family is not always acceptable outside of the family. Children will need to learn how to play co-operatively with their own peers as well as how to interact with adults such as teachers, and playgroup and nursery workers. This will be their first introduction to the rules and expectations of a wider society. They must learn to share, take turns, communicate with children and adults and negotiate their way into games and activities, which is often more complex than just saying 'May I play too'. Having negotiated themselves into a game or activity, children then have to learn and apply the rules that appertain to the situation; those that do not manage to do this will be viewed as spoiling the game. They have to become aware and understand the feelings of others, understanding when they may be hurting other children or being unkind to them. The adult has a large role to play in this as most children learn by

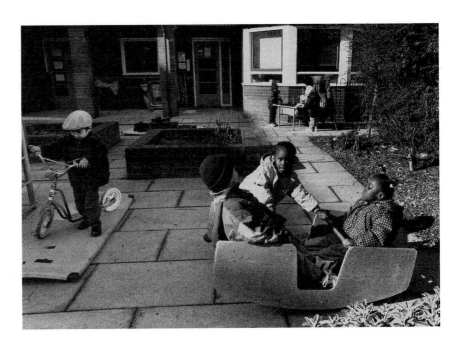

observing and adopting the example offered by the adults around them.

VALUE OF DIFFERENT TYPES OF PLAY

Imaginative Play

This helps children gain pleasure, learn self-expression and explore and solve problems, and enables them to pass from the egocentric stage to objectivity. Pretence and symbolic play are early forms of representation, and fantasy play helps children cope with emotions and problems in childhood.

Fantasy play can start as early as 18 months, but well formed pretend play usually appears around 3 years of age. From the age of 7–8 years, fantasy play begins to diminish as the child's reasoning ability and experience lead them to distinguish between fantasy and reality. However, many adults still appreciate the opportunity to indulge in fantasy play, hence the large number of amateur dramatic societies which flourish around the country. In imaginative play the child rehearses their interests, skills and obligations, and makes experiments in social relationships without having to pay the penalty for mistakes.

Symbolic play enables the child to relive their past experiences, and in older children the symbols are replaced by rules in social play. Role play refers to any activity in which the child assumes a distinct identity different from their own; this is a special category of pretend or make-believe play. In role play the child will announce, 'I am the doctor, Robin is the nurse and Lee is the sick person'. In pretend or make-believe play the child will say, 'I am driving my ambulance to the hospital' whilst they are sitting on a wooden truck.

Dressing-up clothes, cardboard boxes, blocks, household equipment etc. will be the only materials that children will need to indulge in imaginative play. A piece of highly coloured cloth can as easily be used as a sari as it can a bridesmaid dress. Hats and bags are useful items for encouraging make-believe or role play. Role-playing television and film heroes is a very common type of pretend play amongst 4–5-year-olds; they love to indulge in being a superhero for a morning.

As well as aiding social and emotional development, imaginative play develops eye–hand co-ordination and small manipulative skills which are needed to put on and take off clothes, concepts of size and number and sequential order being developed through the play itself. When imaginative play is in groups, social development is aided as children play co-operatively and exchange ideas and take turns in being superheroes.

Constructive/ Manipulative Play

Constructive play enables the child to experience the satisfaction of producing an end product. For the younger child the activity is more important than the end product. Children begin to construct and manipulate materials by using dough, clay, sand, blocks, wood, scissors, paste, crayons etc. They may use their construction as part of their imaginative play. When children first use manipulative play they will not have an end product in mind, although if asked they are likely to make a last-minute decision as to what the construction represents. As they get older and use sophisticated construction toys such as Lego they may have a very definite end product in mind. Older children are capable of producing very complex constructions using blocks, Lego, junk materials etc. Whatever the child produces in their constructive activities must be appreciated and acknowledged by the adult as it would have been made with a lot of thought and effort. Sometimes children will need encouragement to complete a construction and the adult may need to offer suggestions as to how best this can be done. Such a timely intervention may help the child to learn not to opt out when things get difficult. Children can become very absorbed in constructive play and spend long periods of concentration on the activity. Constructive play allows opportunities for solitary, parallel and co-operative play. It is important that the adult does not discourage them; there is nothing more frustrating for the child than being asked to pull apart a construction because it is lunchtime. It is important to have a safe place to keep a half-completed construction so that the child can come back to it after lunch or the next day.

Block Play

The block area should be sited out of the way of traffic in the nursery so that the children can build without interference from others and their construction does not prevent other activities from taking place. The block storage cupboard should be low enough to enable the children to manipulate the blocks in and out of the cupboard and should have sufficient shelves to store blocks of similar shapes together. Large unit blocks allow children to discover equivalences and other mathematical relationships as well as giving children an understanding of space and area.

Block play encourages physical development and the child's gross motor skills as they bend, lift, stretch and crawl. As the child handles each block so they are developing fine muscle control and eye–hand co-ordination. Control of the fingers and hand is seen in the palmar grasp for large blocks and the pincer grasp for the smallest blocks. Balancing on constructions such as 'bridges' promotes foot control, as does standing on tiptoe to reach high blocks.

From blocks, children discover concepts relating to size, shape, position, weight and height. Where the shape of the block is drawn on the shelf to correspond to the position of the block, children are able to relate a two-dimensional drawing with a three-dimensional object as well as learning to identify a block by a symbol. Activities in block play offer the child the opportunity to develop concepts which are the basis of maths, language, physics and social development. Learning that certain blocks stack more easily because they are of a similar shape, a child can stack in a progressive series of size, practise one-to-one correspondence by piling one block onto another, learn that blocks are the parts which go towards making the whole structure of a tower or bridge, and learn how to take away blocks to make a structure lower and how to solve problems. Block play increases a child's vocabulary as they learn the meanings of words such as higher, lower, smaller, larger, skyscraper, factory, bridge, tower etc.

Blocks, as constructive play, enable the child to produce something to their own specifications and this gives them an enormous sense of pride. They develop self-confidence as they learn to manipulate the blocks and get a feeling of satisfaction when they knock down something that they have created. Block play is an activity which allows children to play in groups, sharing ideas, respecting each other's opinions and contributions and problem solving together. It also offers the opportunity for children to play alone, and some days a child will play in a group and other days they will play alone.

Creative Play

Creativity involves discovery, invention, experience, imagination, experimentation, problem solving and establishing new links between what already exists, e.g. a blanket, table and chair can become a cave for exploring. If creativity is to be fostered in the nursery, the attitudes of the staff must allow for children to deviate from the 'norm', as one original piece of work is far more valuable than 20 pieces of work based on an adult-made template. Apart from the obvious creative activities such as painting, collage, junk modelling (see Table 7.1), dough and clay, there are other activities which develop a child's imagination and enable them to express their creativity, activities such as music and movement, dramatic play, dressing up etc. Adventure playgrounds provide scope for free expression and aid development of imagination and creativity with their tyre swings, tree trunks, rope and metal climbing frames, barrels etc.

In using creative materials such as dough, clay and wet sand, the child learns about the properties of natural materials and how these can be manipulated in order to form an end product. They learn about the use of symbols (square for a house, circle for the sun) to represent real objects. The production of pictures and patterns develops the child's aesthetic appreciation. The adult can help develop the child's imagination by extending their experiences with outings, classroom

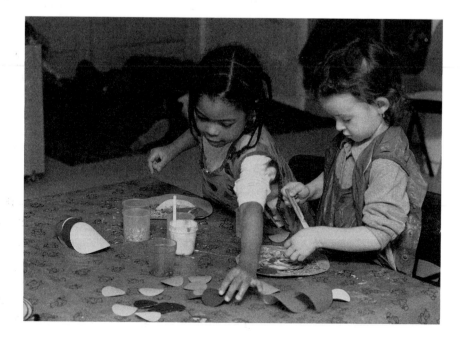

displays, colourful picture books, providing interesting materials such as glittery paper, pieces of exotic material such as silk and satin, corrugated paper, gold and silver foil etc.

Adults should never comment on the artistic value of what the child has produced but must be non-judgemental, appreciating that for the child it is the process that is important and not the product. Every child's work should be put on display, and adults who are skilled at mounting and displaying children's work can make even the poorest effort look splendid.

Table 7.1 Items to collect for the junk table

Aluminium foil	Elastic	Pipe cleaners
Beads	Fablon	Plastic and polystyrene
Birdseed	Feathers	trays
Books	Felt	Plastic bottles
Bottle tops	Fir cones	Polystyrene
Braid	Foam rubber	Raffia
Brushes	Foil dishes	Ribbon
Buttons	Fringes	Rice
Candles	Glitter	Sand
Cardboard	Grasses (dried)	Sawdust (can be coloured
Cards (birthday,	Ice lolly sticks	with food colouring or
Christmas, holiday)	Insulating tape	powder paint)
Cartons	Jewellery	Seeds
Cereal packs (cut to give	Kitchen roll centres	Sequins
a good solid base)	Lace	Sheep's wool
Cellophane (off sweets,	Leather	Shells
etc.)	Leaves	Shoe boxes
Chalk	Lino (scrap)	Silver paper
Cheese boxes	Lolly sticks	Squeezy bottles
Christmas paper	Magazines (for cutting	Straw
Coat hangers	out)	String
Cocktail sticks	Margarine containers	Sweet papers
Coloured paper	Match boxes	Tape
Corks	Material (scrap)	Threads
Corrugated paper	Meat trays	Tiles (ceiling)
Cotton reels	Melon seeds	Tissue boxes
Cotton wool	Milk bottle tops	Trimmings, e.g. lace,
Crayons	Net bags	braid, ric-rac
Doilies	Netting	Velcro
Dried:	Newspapers	Wallpaper (rolls and old
coffee granules	Nut shells	books)
egg shells	Paper	Wood
melon seeds	Paper plates and cups	Wood shavings
sand	Pebbles	Wool (used and new)
tea leaves	Pine cones	Yoghurt cartons
Egg cartons	Ping pong balls	

In painting and creative activities, children develop fine muscle control through management of the brush, using different parts of the body to paint with (e.g. foot painting) and controlling the amount of paint that they will use. The child is able to make decisions as to where on the paper they will start, what the end product will be, or what character they will dress up as. They will experiment with paint mixing colours together, they will try modelling with wet and dry sand and learn that you cannot model with dry clay. Children get great enjoyment from this experimentation process; it can be very satisfying for a child to find out what it is like to walk in high-heeled shoes or wear a wig. Through creative activities a child can express themselves, particularly releasing strong feelings when slapping paint on paper, banging dough, hammering wood and nails. These activities allow a child to work at their own pace, either alone or with others.

Stages of development in children's painting

Rhoda Kellogg (1955) carried out studies of children's drawing in Africa, Japan, Tonga, Austria and England, and found that all children react to paint in the same way. If given something to draw with and something to draw on they will discover by themselves and then use similar drawing symbols. Patterns of development are clearly seen in the universality of the symbols which they use and the order in which they use them. It does not matter at what age a child has their first experience of drawing, they will go through the same development

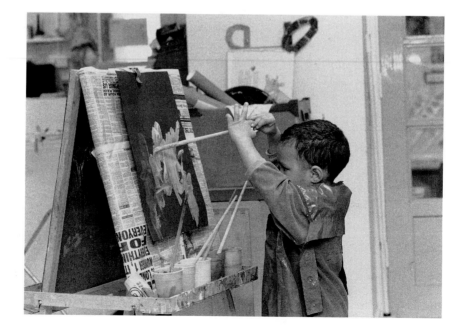

stages using the same symbols. Obviously for an older child with greater muscle control many of these stages will be passed through very quickly.

Almost all children begin drawing by scribbling and as Jameson (1973) points out, they may use any medium to do this, 'fingers in food, sticks in dust or sand, steam on the window, but they soon graduate to more positive media like crayons, chalk, pencil on blackboard or wall paper in the sitting room or . . . large sketch books or pads.' They will continue to scribble until they move towards a shape, usually an oval. The child then develops the oval into a house, a cat, a bird, anything they want to develop it into. From the oval the child develops what Jameson describes as the radial; this is where the child has added radii coming out from the oval. Children begin to use the oval as the head and the radii as arms and legs (not necessarily in the correct numbers). In order to develop the head the child will add dots in a circle for eyes, a mouth depicted by a line of scribble and a circle on each side of the oval to depict ears. The number of radii diminish so there are two representing legs and sometimes there will also be two for arms. The child will use this figure for playing out fantasies and symbolizing their experiences. The next stage of development is when the child begins to experiment with paint. The first stage is when the child makes blobs of colour on the paper indicating that they have found the paint and are manipulating the paint and brush to connect with the paper. They find they can create different colours by mixing one on top of the other on the paper. They then discover that by using each individual brush that is in each pot of paint or washing their brush before going to a new colour they can create more distinct colours which resemble colours in the environment. They learn to manipulate the brush from scribble movements, to dots, to patches. They will fill the whole paper with patches of colour. In order to do this, children need skill and co-ordination, and need to make choices. They will aesthetically superimpose one colour on top of another in order to create colourful patterns. They will become more controlled in their application of colour, sequencing colours and shapes. The next stage is when they connect the use of paint and their drawings of the oval and radii to produce what Jameson describes as a colourful 'big head'. They use this to symbolize their experiences. The 'big head' then moves through arms and legs to them adding a body by using a patch of colour. The body then may be given arms, the head will be given hair and by around 5 years of age they will be painting fingers at the ends of arms and toes or shoes at the ends of legs. Once they have become confident in drawing the figure they will progress to painting the 'house'. This starts out as an empty square with patches of colour for the windows. They will slowly add new symbols to the house, e.g. squares for window glass, a chimney and a door, so that the painting of the house becomes more sophisticated and complex. They may even add the sun, rain, trees, or turn the house into a caravan by giving it wheels. They will also give complicated explanations of their paintings, often telling the adult the story attached to the symbols. By the age of 6–7 years their drawings have become quite detailed and sophisticated with large buildings, many people, cars, aeroplanes, cats, dogs, rainbows, snow etc. and there is evidence of a lot of activity happening in the pictures. Their paintings represent the things which they have seen around them or may be part of a project such as dinosaurs, zoo animals etc.

Books and Storytelling

Children's knowledge and creative thinking are encouraged and developed by books and stories. Children not only get a great deal of enjoyment from books but they also benefit emotionally, intellectually, socially, linguistically and culturally. Feely books can offer young children tactile experiences as can books made of different materials such as cardboard, cloth, plastic inflatable floatable books etc. For very young children, books should have large clear illustrations of familiar objects or animals in primary colours, with no or few written words. Pictures must be complete, cars must have four wheels and animals

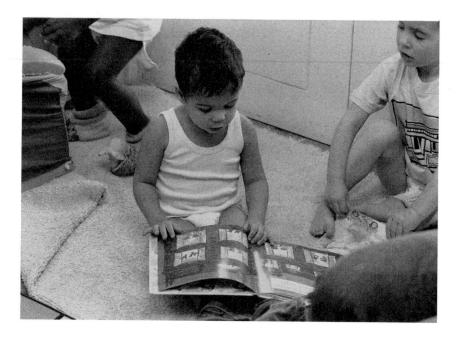

must have a head, body and four legs. At this age, books are to look at and the adult can talk to the child about the pictures in the book; it is not necessary to have a story line.

For a child it is a pleasant emotional experience to be sat on an adult's lap looking at a book while the adult reads the story. The child feels safe and secure and they like to ask for their favourite story to be read over and over again. In the school or nursery there should be a book corner which should appear warm and inviting with a carpet, low shelves so that the children can reach the books and small comfortable chairs. Storytime can take place in the book corner with the adult reading to a small group of children. Books and stories teach children to sit still for a short period of time, develop concentration, practise language and learn new words, experience emotions such as joy, excitement and fear, and share experiences with others, e.g. going to the dentist, getting a new brother or sister. Books are able to make the connections for the child, between the symbol (picture) and the written word and the spoken word. Books are also informational, giving extra and exciting details about things seen on outings, in the shops, in the garden etc. The child's curiosity is stimulated to ask questions, and the adult can help the child to find answers from books.

The book corner should be in a quiet area of the room, it should be warm, well lit and comfortable. Books should be displayed attractively in a purpose-built display rack, which could be homemade. The books on display should be changed regularly. Many nurseries and schools have a system whereby children can take a book home overnight so they can read it with their parents. All the children must understand that the book corner is a quiet area of the room and that it is not the place for noisy or boisterous play. Children must be taught to handle books carefully, to respect them so that they can be shared by all the children. Any torn books should be mended straightaway, if possible making sure that the child that did the tearing is involved in the repairing. Old, tattered, dog-eared books should be removed as they will not be attractive to the children. Books should have pictures which reflect children from different cultures, different family styles, males and females in non-stereotypical roles. Books need to be very carefully chosen to ensure that they are not giving children the wrong messages about race, culture and equal opportunities.

Specialist suppliers like the Letter Box Library are able to provide lists of non-racist, non-sexist books for children (address at the back of the book). Pop-up books are not suitable for group usage as they very easily get torn and look unattractive.

Traditional stories such as 'The Three Little Pigs', 'Billy Goats

Gruff' and 'Tale of a Turnip' are popular, as they have a lot of repetition that the children like to join in. There are also translations of traditional Asian and Afro-Caribbean stories such as 'Anansi the Spider' which are popular with children. Informational books should be colourful and have good clear illustrations. These books may become part of a display on the interest table. It is also useful to have a large picture encyclopaedia to enable the children to look up information about any topic they are particularly interested in.

When reading stories to children make sure that they are all sitting comfortably, that they can all see the book. Hold the book open and face the children as you read the story. Stop to point to illustrations or to ask the children questions. Read slowly and clearly with animation so that the children's interest is held. A good storyteller will be able to alter their voice to indicate excitement, fear, different characters in the story etc. It is essential for the adult to have read the story themselves before they read it to the children; this way they will become familiar with the story and be able to read it in a more animated way.

Storytelling was a custom long before books were written and was often a way of passing on oral history and information. A story can be told without a book but it may be a version of a story in a book or it can be a total original story. Props such as puppets, bags and hats can be used to enliven the story. As in reading a story, the teller must adopt different voices for different characters and use their voice to express emotions. Telling stories well requires imagination and advance preparation on the part of the storyteller.

Children love rhymes and poetry as they enjoy the repetition and learn to join in. Action rhymes such as 'Miss Polly had a Dolly' are very popular, with children being able to play the different roles. Counting rhymes may help children to learn numbers, although much of this may be learning by rote as most of the rhymes require the child to count backwards! Stories told in rhyme have a great appeal to children, particularly if they are also ring games such as 'There was a Lovely Princess', which is the story of Sleeping Beauty in rhyme. The poems of AA Milne are very popular with older children (6–7 years) and may encourage children to write their own poetry. The basis of all poetry is the flow and rhythm of the language used, described by Coleridge as 'the best words in the best order', therefore they are a very early introduction to children of rhythm.

Music, Movement, Dance

Children can be introduced to musical sounds from a very early age; there are musical mobiles available which can be suspended over the baby's cot. Children like to create their own musical sounds, even babies enjoy the tinkle of bells or the sound of the rattle. Adults sing to children and will play music to them from an early age. The lullaby is traditionally a calming quiet song which will soothe a baby. As children get older they can express their emotions through playing musical instruments or participating in music and movement. Music develops children's listening skills, trains their ear to distinguish between different musical instruments and introduces them to rhythms. Through music and movement sessions they are able to learn to control both large and small muscles, learn body co-ordination and move in time to the music. It also offers the opportunity for self-expression and creativity as they find a way to 'be a wave in a stormy sea' or 'be an elephant'. Most nurseries have a music area where different instruments are displayed. It is not necessary to purchase expensive instruments, as homemade shakers, bells, drums, tambourines, cymbals, gongs, recorders etc. will be all that is needed. Instruments from other cultures such as castanets, skin drums, pan pipes and bamboo pipes will broaden the children's knowledge and experience. Children can experiment with these, finding out what type of noise each makes and how they work, whether they are plucked, blown, shaken or banged. Children are able to clap out simple rhythmic patterns in songs, poems or music. Music can be used to calm feelings or express emotions; a good bang on a drum can release a lot of frustration.

Music also aids the development of children's listening skills. They have to learn to listen to music and other sounds around them. If you are going to clap in rhythm to the music then you must listen to the music. If you are going to sing accompanied by a piano or guitar then you must listen to the notes played on the instrument. Children should be introduced to a wide variety of music using tapes, CDs or records; this is also an opportunity to play music from other cultures so that they get a broad view of what music is about. When children make their own music this can be tape-recorded and played back to them so they are able to listen to their own product.

Scenario 7.2

Your Officer-in-Charge has given you a budget of £200 to restock the book corner in your nursery room. The room caters for children between the ages of 3–4 years. Draw up a list of criteria that you will use in order to select the books.

Water Play

This can be an indoor or outdoor activity or could be helping the adult to wash up or wash clothes. The earliest form of water play for children is bath time. In the nursery there will be a purpose-made water trolley which is usually equipped with a large variety of pipes, tubes, sieves, plastic bottles, jugs, waterwheel, corks, wood, rock etc. Through their experimental and exploratory play with water, children learn about the properties of water, conservation of volume, sinking and floating, bubbles and water as a source of power to turn a wheel. These are all early scientific concepts. If water play is outside on a hot summer day, they will also learn that the heat is able to dry spilt water and that the water gets warm in the heat. Water play is made more interesting by varying the equipment and colouring the water.

The child care worker needs to ask children questions which extend their understanding of the basic concepts and allow them to problem solve, for example 'What happens if you fill one big jug with water, is there enough water to fill two small jugs?' 'Let's find out which of these toys sink and which float.' 'What happens to water if it's put into the freezer?'

Playing with water can prove to be a very relaxing activity for children and adults. Water satisfies all the senses; it makes a lovely sound, it looks inviting and on a hot day a refreshing drink of clean cool water is welcomed. Water is a very versatile medium for children to use and they can repeat experiments over and over again. Most children like water, splashing in puddles, bath time, going to the paddling pool, watching ships, going to the seaside are pleasurable activities. There is a lot to find out about water, particularly when it is ice or snow. Water play can be a solitary activity or a co-operative activity, for example a group of children decide to wash dolls' clothes and bath dolls and do this together. Water play leads to a lot of communication between children and between adults and children.

Sand Play

Once again sand is a good medium for understanding scientific concepts such as flowing, gritty, moulding etc. Most nurseries and playgroups have a sand trolley. Sand play needs to offer children both wet and dry sand, as the concepts of each are different. Children like to bury things in sand and then rediscover these objects at a later point. Children can draw in wet sand and watch the picture disappear as the sand dries out, they can also draw a picture on paper using glue and then sprinkle dry sand over this.

As with water play, the role of the adult is one of extending the children's understanding and thinking and introducing them to the language which goes with the concepts. Questions such as 'What does dry sand feel like?' 'Which type of sand goes through the sieve the

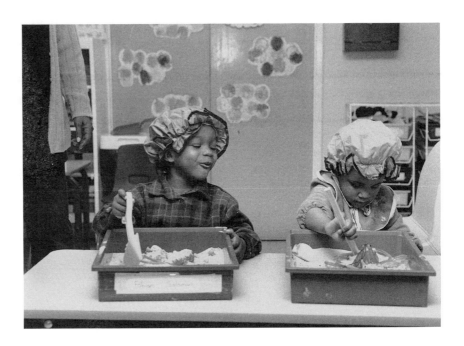

fastest, wet or dry?' 'Are there any things which are the same about sand and water?'. Older children are able to make sand and water clocks to compare these likenesses and differences. Sand can be used indoors and outside; often outside there is a large sandpit which gives great scope for building large tunnels, castles and other structures. Sand play can be both a solitary activity and co-operative activity. It does not have the same soothing effect upon children as water play but it can prove to be just as exciting.

Playing with Clay

Clay is another natural material that children like to play with. They will discover that it is more difficult to mould than dough and requires a lot of rolling, kneading and banging to get into shape. Children do not need a lot of equipment to play with clay, just a board and rolling pin, the rest they can do with their hands. Children's products can be kept and dried (there is clay available which does not need firing) and then the children can paint them. Clay play is usually a solitary activity although children may be given a specific task such as moulding 'cakes' to go in the home corner or class shop or making animals to go into the farm area or forming three-dimensional shapes for maths. Clay, because it needs a great deal of strength to mould, is not suitable for very young children; it is better to give them dough.

The role of the adult is very important in the storing of clay as it dries out very easily and is then unable to be used. Most nurseries will have a plastic clay bin which has a tight fitting lid, the clay is stored in this but first needs to be wrapped in a damp cloth and then placed in a plastic bag. Older children will be able to help the adult do this and understand the relationship between water and clay. Clay play is a very good medium for boisterous children to use in order to work out their aggression and excess energy.

Scenario 7.3

Gemma is 4 years old and at times is inclined to be disruptive. Today Gemma has torn three books in the book corner. How do you handle this situation so that Gemma develops a greater understanding of the way books should be treated?

Cooking/Preparing Food

Older children love to participate in cooking or other food preparation activities. Cooking is a co-operative activity which is done in small groups and requires an adult to plan, lead and oversee the children to ensure safety. It is an excellent learning medium, starting with a visit to the shops to buy the required ingredients and ending with the children eating or taking home their products. Not all food activities require a cooker, for example, making ice lollies, making sandwiches, cold sweets which are made from whisking substances into milk or making jellies.

From a cookery session, children will learn a great deal of science and maths, how heat changes substances, thickening through whisking, the effects of extreme cold on substances, weighing, counting different things in different ways e.g. eggs counted singly, flour weighed, flavourings in teaspoons or drops etc. Children will also learn how to listen to and carry out instructions, how to work together to weigh, mix, stir and knead, and how to share out the end product. They will also learn the beginnings of food hygiene, washing hands, cleaning the table, wearing an apron, how to treat knives with respect, cleaning up after them whilst the food is cooking. Different types of vegetables and fruit can be introduced and these can be explored by cutting them in half, peeling them and tasting them raw and cooked; they may even grow their own vegetables such as mustard and cress and then make sandwiches with it for lunch.

Language is developed by naming ingredients, utensils, cooking terms (e.g. roll, knead, chop and grate), mathematical language (e.g. grammes, litres, and kilos), and scientific language (e.g. boiling, roasting, baking, melting and freezing), which will all be explored in cookery. For some children who may live in a home where microwaved dinners are the norm, cooking can be a totally new experience. It is also a good time for the adult to talk to the children about healthy eating and introducing foods from different cultures; this is an area where you may be able to involve parents in demonstrating different cooking utensils such as woks, paella pans etc. Cooking is an all-round

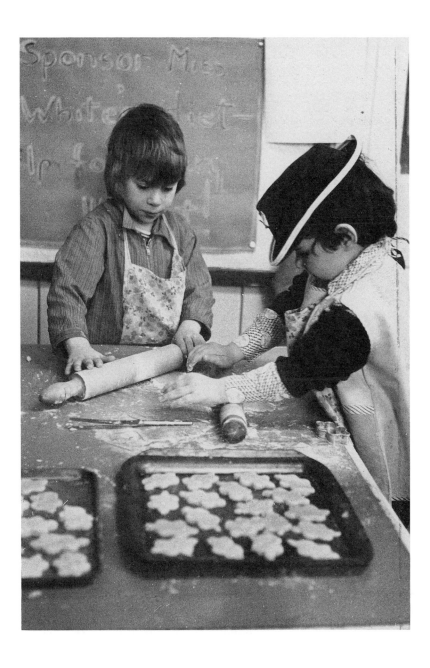

intensive learning situation, but is such an exciting activity that children are always more than willing to participate.

Interest Tables

Most nurseries and schools have an interest table which is changed on a regular basis. The interest table may be based on a particular theme, such as 'weather', 'cats' or 'mini-beasts', or maybe teaching children a particular concept, such as colours or numbers. The whole idea of an interest table is to bring together items which the children can examine, explore and discuss with the adult and each other. It must look attractive; a few carefully chosen items are better than a packed table. All the items displayed must be safe for the children to touch and explore (no rough edges, sharp points, non-toxic, not precious or irreplaceable etc.). The staff team will usually decide on the themes for the interest table, and the staff may take it in turns to be responsible for themes. The interest table should also have informational books which are open at the appropriate pages, along with pictures, photographs or other illustrations. When the interest table is first set up, the children's attention should be drawn to it and it should be explained to them what it is about and how they can use it. This should be done each time that the theme is changed. Sometimes children will bring in additional items for the table and these should be put on display. Flowers and plants may be displayed and it is important to involve the children in watering and caring for them; however, children should be discouraged from picking flowers and plants to bring into school as they could be poisonous, and it is not in line with present thinking about conservation.

SETTING OUT AND CLEARING AWAY PLAY ACTIVITIES

It is the adult's responsibility to plan and organize play activities for children. The usual method of doing this is through a team meeting of all the staff who are working with the children. The school or nursery may have long-term aims and objectives for the children and the activities will need to ensure that they enable the children to reach these aims. For example, the aim for the next month is to encourage the children's concept development in maths and science and to extend their language, the theme may be 'the weather', therefore all activities for the next 2 weeks will start from the weather. In addition to this there may be specific learning goals for certain children who may have special needs or behaviour problems.

Planning

A weekly meeting of the team will decide on the activities and the specific responsibilities of each member of staff. Certain equipment is likely to be on hand every day for the children such as water, sand, painting, dressing up, home corner etc.; however, it will probably be necessary to vary the equipment in each of these areas so that it fits in with the learning outcomes. For example, using the weather theme the dressing-up corner would have mackintoshes, umbrellas, scarves, hats, coats, gloves, sunshades, dark glasses etc.; the water trolley will have sprays, waterproof materials and ice; the cookery session will make hot things for cold days and cool drinks for hot days. Part of the planning may require some children going to the shops or on a small outing elsewhere. It is important to ensure that there is parental permission for this type of activity and the adult needs to decide when they will go, who they will take, where they will go, what the purpose of the visit is and that there are enough adults to adequately supervise the number of children. Once the plans for the week have been made and each member of staff has been allocated their particular areas of responsibility the plans should then be displayed on the inside of a cupboard door to ensure that everyone is aware of what everyone else is doing. This is particularly important if you are a candidate on placement as you may only be at the nursery for 2 days a week, but whatever you will be doing on those days needs to be communicated to all staff so that there is no duplication or confusion.

Setting Out Equipment

The adult's most important role in setting out activities is to ensure that they are in a position that is safe for the children. You may also need to consider access for children with special needs. Activities need to be kept well away from doors and main walkways.

The room should be set up well in advance of the children arriving. In many cases there is not a lot of alteration that can be done to the layout of the room. For example, the water trolley has a permanent spot close to the bathroom, the shop has replaced the home corner for a number of weeks, the quiet area/book corner is in a fixed position; the only features which may be open to movement are the tables. However, you can do quite a lot with tables, joining a number together for a large junk modelling activity or deciding whether the optimum number should be two or four children playing with the Lego etc. When putting out table toys it is important to think about the practicalities; if the Lego is always ending up in the sand trolley then make sure that it is on a table as far away from the sand as possible. Remember the stages of development of the children and ensure that there are activities available that offer progressive complexity as well as those that are easy. There must be enough space for the children to walk easily around the tables and enough space on the table for the number of participants to be able to play freely.

The equipment should look attractive to the children; this means no puzzles with missing pieces, attractive containers for Lego and Duplo, fresh paint and clean brushes, clean paper on the easels, clay that has not dried out, dressing-up clothes that are clean and displayed on hangers. Always make sure that you have protective aprons for water play, painting, clay and cooking, and allow the right number of aprons for the number of children participating in the activity. During the activities it is important to mop up any spillages quickly and ensure that there is always clean paper for painting, and fresh dough or clay when children change activity. Children should not have to re-use another child's leftover material; they should all have equal opportunity to use fresh materials.

Clearing Away Activities and Storing Equipment

Wherever possible the children should be involved in clearing away equipment as this is good training for them; however, this must be done in a safe way. Small equipment should be stored in clearly labelled boxes or trays on shelves or tray racks. Any products that the children wish to keep should be put in a safe place until home time. Paintings should be labelled with the child's name and pegged up to dry. Tables should be wiped down, dried and stacked in a safe place; do not get children to help in moving furniture. Jigsaws and matching games should be checked to ensure that all the pieces are complete. Paint pots should be cleaned or securely lidded if they are to be re-used, and brushes must be washed and left to dry. Aprons must be washed and hung up to dry. Equipment should be regularly checked for safety and wear. Any equipment which needs mending should be removed from the play area and reported to the appropriate person. Outdoor equipment needs to be checked for rust and that nuts and bolts are not coming loose. Movable outdoor equipment should be kept in a locked shed, and sand pits should have a purpose-built cover to prevent cats and other animals polluting the sand.

EARLY YEARS CURRICULUM

The early years curriculum has been the subject of debate for many years and now few would deny that there is a range of learning opportunities offered to children in the pre-school years which can be defined in curriculum terms. Curtis (1986) stated,

> . . . there is a recognizable curriculum for children under statutory school age based on skills and competencies to be developed in a flexible and child-centred environment, and there is ample

material with which to challenge and extend children without offering them a 'watered down' reception class programme.

The Rumbold Committee (DES, 1990) looked into the educational experiences offered to 3- and 4-year-olds, and in its report *Starting with Quality* defines the curriculum as follows:

> The curriculum – which we take to comprise the concepts, knowledge, understanding, attitudes and skills that a child needs to develop – can be defined and expressed in a number of different ways. These varying approaches include frameworks based on subjects, resource areas, broad themes or areas of learning.

The Rumbold report gives the areas of learning which go towards constructing a curriculum for the under-fives as:

◆ Aesthetic and creative
◆ Human and social
◆ Language and literacy
◆ Mathematics
◆ Physical
◆ Science
◆ Spiritual and moral
◆ Technology

Rumbold goes into great detail regarding the contents and activities which come under each of these headings. However, the following is a concise version which is taken from a document produced by ILEA (1987):

> *Aesthetic and creative:* about symbolic representation, imaginative play, art and craft work, display, drama, movement and music. About doing their own creations and appreciating the creations of others.

> *Human and social:* about how we live and the world of work, about relationships with each other and the environment. About actions in the past and their relationship to the present and future. About physical and human conditions.

> *Language and literacy:* about symbolic representation and about listening, talking, reading and writing.

> *Mathematics:* about recognizing and solving problems, about sorting and classifying and identifying relationships and patterns. About pure numbers, measures, logic and sets and their application to other areas.

Physical: about body awareness, co-ordination and control, about spatial, manipulative and motor skills. About imaginative use of the body, about health and its maintenance.

Scientific and technological: about problem solving, about changing and controlling the environment. About ourselves and living things, about physical surroundings, about forces, movement and energy.

Moral: about awareness of self and others, about right and wrong, fairness and justice. About being a member of a group and wider community.

Spiritual: about significance of life, about sense of awe and wonder, about myths and legends. About religious experiences reflecting many faiths.

There have been in existence for some time a number of curricula models; some are based upon the theories of the well known educators upon whose philosophies they depend and others have developed for differing reasons. Four of these will be looked at in detail: Highscope, Steiner, Montessori and Portage.

Highscope

This was first introduced in the USA in the 1960s as part of the Head Start programme. Head Start was a Federal initiative put into place to reduce the educational disadvantage of children from socially and economically deprived backgrounds. Highscope was introduced to the UK in the mid-1980s. Highscope programmes encourage children to be problem solvers and decision makers, and to attain independence through a framework of activities. It places special emphasis on children planning their own activities and then reflection upon how the activity went; this is known as Plan–Do–Review. A typical Highscope day would be broken into: greeting, planning time, work time, clean up time, recall time, circle time, small group time, outside time, end of session and recording, when the adults write up their account of each child. Highscope materials clearly define what each child should be doing and also what each adult's role should be during the activity. From this point of view the Highscope method is highly structured.

Rudolf Steiner (1861–1925)

The methods based upon the philosophy of Steiner are referred to as the Waldorf education system. Steiner believed that childhood existed as a period of life in its own right and he was concerned about developing all the characteristics of the growing child. The Waldorf curriculum aims to give the child a balanced experience of arts and sciences, balance in the processes of thinking, feeling and willing. It seeks to educate more than just the intellect, giving the child open options to learn. The environment of the nursery is very important and must provide a warm joyful atmosphere. The day may begin with a circle activity and singing games. Children are free to play with others or alone. Play is usually with natural materials, there are no manufactured toys or games. There are seasonal decorations such as leaves, twigs, pine cones, stones, crystals, rocks etc. There are numerous wooden blocks of different sizes, textures and shapes. Imaginative play is a central activity in the Waldorf system. The role of the teacher is to be ready to help or join in. The teacher is leader, instigator and role model as they have the task of firing the children's imaginations by telling stories (not reading stories), singing songs, playing games, pointing out things in the natural world, painting alongside the children, baking, sewing etc. The teacher must be well prepared and a good role model for the children to imitate.

Maria Montessori (1869–1952)

Montessori's philosophy is based upon enabling each child to develop to their full potential. She believed that children's minds are able to absorb complex concepts about the world around them in an effortless way. She saw children learning through observation, exploration and movement. Montessori nursery schools are meant to be a homely environment with different areas for quiet activities, table work, floor activities and free access to a garden. Children have the freedom to choose what they wish to do and spend as long as they need on an activity. Independence and self-motivation are encouraged. They work with specially designed equipment which enables the child to make discoveries about the world around them. The adult's role is to involve themselves by working alongside the child, to prepare the environment to enable children to learn spontaneously, to act as a link between the child and the materials and to observe the children. As they observe the children they take notes and decide which materials should be presented to the child next in order for them to progress to the next development stage.

Portage

This a system which was devised in the USA. It is a structured home-based programme to teach children skills and is most useful for children with special needs or developmental delay. Portage is delivered by specially trained people who may be teachers, health workers or volunteers. The Portage worker negotiates with parents/carers as to which skills will be taught to the child. The parents/carers are responsible for repeating the programme with the child between the visits of the Portage worker and for recording the progress of the child. The Portage package consists of teaching cards, activity charts and checklists which cover infant stimulation, socialization, self-help, language, cognitive and motor skills. It is a very highly structured system with each task broken down into small steps, each step being slightly more complex than the preceding step. Because it is very structured it works best with parents/carers who are highly motivated and well organized. Although the aim of the Portage system is predominantly to benefit the child, it often leads to parents/carers having a better understanding of the child and helps them to develop more confidence in working with the child.

OBSERVATION AND ASSESSMENT

A feature of all early years curricula is that there should be an element of observation and assessment of the child in order to record the child's progress. Information on the abilities of the child is useful for the parents, the school and the child's developmental records. Teachers and child care workers are able to plan a programme of future activities for children if they are aware of the developmental stages the children have reached and the competences that they already have. Certain children may need extra help or need to spend longer on specific activities. The responsibility for undertaking and recording assessment usually lies with the teacher, the nursery officer or the most senior person working with a group of children. However, all staff are able to make contributions by carrying out observations on groups of children or target children. Observing children is a basic skill needed by all those who are intending to work with children. It is a skill which can be developed through training and practised 'on the job'. Confidentiality is an important aspect of observation and assessment, and any observations which are going to be used for purposes outside of the placement must ensure that the child remains anonymous or the parents/guardians have given permission for the observation to be used.

LEARNING OUTCOMES FOR PRE-SCHOOL CHILDREN

More recently the emphasis has moved away from the curriculum and moved towards learning outcomes. Learning outcomes are what a child can be expected to do at a certain stage in development or by a certain age, whereas the curriculum is concerned with the activities which will produce the learning outcomes. At the time of this book going to press the 'Desirable Outcomes for Children's Learning on Entering Compulsory Education' (DFEE, 1996b) have just been published by the Department for Education and Employment. These are the goals for learning which children should have reached by the time they enter compulsory education, i.e. the term after the child is 5 years of age. It is expected that prior to entering school all children, but particularly 4-year-olds, should pursue a curriculum which enables them to progress towards the learning outcomes. To enable all 4-year-olds to participate the present government intends issuing vouchers to parents; these will cover five sessions per week for the child in a pre-school establishment. Therefore playgroups, nursery schools,

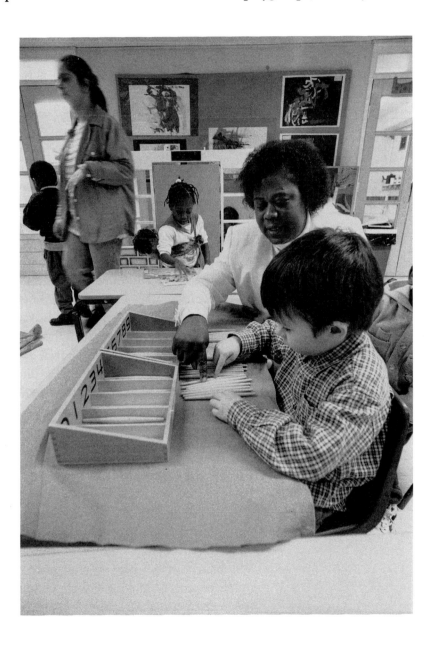

combined nursery centres and other early years establishments will be devising a curriculum for the 3–5-year-olds which will enable children to work towards the desirable outcomes. The six areas of learning are as follows: personal and social development, language and literacy, mathematics, knowledge and understanding of the world, physical development and creative development. Examples of some of the learning outcomes under these headings are as follows:

◆ *Personal and social development.* Children are confident, are able to establish relationships with other children and adults, work as part of a group and independently, are able to concentrate, are eager to explore, initiate ideas, solve simple problems, are sensitive to the feelings of others

◆ *Language and literacy.* Children listen attentively, talk about their experiences, use a growing vocabulary, listen and respond to stories, rhymes, poems and songs, make up their own stories, enjoy books, recognize their own name, recognize letters of the alphabet

◆ *Mathematics.* Children use mathematical language, recognize and create patterns, compare, sort, match, order, count, recognize and use numbers up to 10

◆ *Knowledge and understanding of the world.* Children talk about where they live, their families and events in their lives, recognize features of living things, use technology where appropriate

◆ *Physical development.* Children move confidently and imaginatively, develop increasing control and co-ordination, use large and small equipment, use balancing and climbing apparatus

◆ *Creative development.* Children explore sound and colour, texture and shape in two and three dimensions, show ability to use imagination through art, music, dance, stories, use a wide range of materials and suitable tools

PARENTS AS PARTNERS

The DFEE (1996a,b) highlights the very influential role that parents/primary carers have upon the learning achievements of the child. The home experiences of the child are significant and will be reflected in the child's learning at nursery or school. It is therefore important that child care workers acknowledge this influence and work in partnership with parents. Braun (1992) points out that there is a failure on the part of child care workers to recognize just how much parents achieve for their children; this failure is seen through the negative attitudes which many workers have towards parents. Braun (1992) believes that most parents have the highest aspirations for their children, although they may lack resources and information as to how these aspirations may be met. Involving parents in their children's care and education will give them confidence and this has very positive spin-offs for the child.

Scenario 7.4

Chen Lee is 4 years old and has just started at your nursery school. On his first day at school, his mother, Mrs Chen, was very reluctant to stay with him. Draw up a programme of how you could best make a relationship with Mrs Chen and encourage her to participate in her son's learning.

Pugh and De'Ath (1989) put forward 10 key factors that can help or hinder partnerships with parents and about which the establishment must make decisions and implement policies. Braun (1992) offers a shorter list of ways in which parents/families can be involved:

(1) there might be space set aside, such as a parents' room where parents can meet or drop in for a chat to one another;
(2) parents or other family members might be used as helpers – in regular group activities, or less regularly, on trips;
(3) specific provision might be made, e.g. parent and toddler group or parenting groups aimed to support parents in their role;
(4) particular attention might be focused on communications at the beginning and end of a session, when families are leaving and then collecting children;
(5) parents can be involved in the management of the service, through membership of its governing body or management committee.

Parents must be made to feel welcome and there should be opportunities for them to participate in activities, exchange information with the child care workers, meet other parents and be informed of their child's progress. They should also be given information about the curriculum and ways in which they can help their child. Parents from ethnic groups may like to be invited to tell the children stories, rhymes or music from their culture or explain about their foods and demonstrate ethnic cooking utensils. Some parents may find it difficult to become involved in this way as they may be working or studying full time, may feel embarrassed or be shy, or they may not feel that they have an adequate command of English if this is not their first language. Braun (1992) points out that child care staff often confuse a parent's non-involvement with disinterest rather than taking time to find the real reasons. The first starting point in forming a relationship is to have respect for parents, listen to what they have to say and not to make assumptions about people.

Relationships should be developed remembering that they are important for the child whose welfare is paramount for the parent and the child care worker. Staff should not let their own attitudes and values exert an influence on relationships with parents. Many establishments have a particular member of staff who is responsible for liaison with parents; this person may have had training in dealing with parents and would need to be a very good communicator. Parents have a right to know the mission statement of the establishment, the curriculum and how they will be informed of their children's progress before they make a decision to send their child to that nursery, playgroup or school. Parents would wish to know that the establishment that their child will attend will not be in conflict with their own values, religion or culture.

Assignments

1. Write an essay on the value of play for the child.

2. Draw a plan of a nursery room showing the layout of activities that will be available for the children. Give reasons for your choice of layout.

3. Write a plan for a cookery session for a group of six 3-year-olds. Give full explanations of the choice of recipe, how you will organize the session and what you expect the children to learn from the session.

4. Undertake the following observations and evaluate each observation in the light of your knowledge of child development and learning:

(a) A 2½-year-old playing with dry sand
(b) A 3-year-old playing in the dressing-up corner
(c) A music and movement session for a group of 4-year-olds
(d) A 5-year-old painting

5. What special adaptations might you need to make in order to enable a 4-year-old with spina bifida, who has a wheelchair, to gain full access to all indoor play activities?

6. Write an introductory booklet for parents telling them about your nursery, the curriculum, how they will receive information on their child's progress and the opportunities for parental involvement.

REFERENCES AND FURTHER READING

Athey, Chris (1990). *Extending Thought in Young Children: a parent teacher partnership*. Paul Chapman, London.

Bee, Helen (1992) *The Developing Child*, p. 323. Harper Collins, New York.

Braun, Dorit (1992). Working with parents. In *Contemporary Issues in the Early Years* (Ed. Gillian Pugh). NCB/Paul Chapman, London.

Brierley, John (1987). *Give me a Child Until he is Seven: brain studies and early childhood education*. Falmer Press, London.

Britton, Lesley (1992). *Montessori Play and Learn*. Vermilion, London.

Bruce, Tina (1989). *Early Childhood Education*. Hodder & Stoughton, Sevenoaks.

Bruce, Tina (1991). *Time To Play in Early Childhood Education*. Hodder & Stoughton, Sevenoaks.

Buddulph, Liz and McQueen, Diana (1995). *How To Help Talking*. First Community Health NHS Trust, Cannock, Staffs.

Curtis, Audrey (1986). *A Curriculum for the Pre-school Child: learning to learn*. NFER-Nelson, Windsor.

David, Tricia (1992). Curriculum in the early years. In *Contemporary Issues in the Early Years* (ed. Gillian Pugh). NCB/Paul Chapman, London.

Department of Health (1993). The Rights of the Child: a guide to the UN Convention. HMSO, London.

Derman-Sparks, Louise (1989). *Anti-bias Curriculum: Tools for empowering young children*. NAEYC, Washington DC.

DES (1990). *Starting with Quality: Report of the Committee of Inquiry into the Quality of the Educational Experience offered to 3–4 year olds*. HMSO, London.

DFEE (1996a). *Nursery Education Scheme: the next steps*. HMSO, London.

DFEE (1996b). *Nursery Education: desirable outcomes for children's learning on entering compulsory education*. HMSO, London.

Drummond, Mary Jane, Lally, Margaret and Pugh, Gillian (1989). *Developing a Curriculum for the Early Years*. National Children's Bureau, London.

Drummond, Mary Jane and Nutbrown, Cathy (1992). Observing and assessing young children. In *Contemporary Issues in the Early Years* (ed. Gillian Pugh). NCB/Paul Chapman, London.

Hurst, Victoria (1991). *Planning for Early Learning: education in the first 5 years*. Paul Chapman, London.

ILEA (1987). *The Early Years: a curriculum for young children*. ILEA Learning Resources Branch, London.

Isaacs, Susan (1954). *The Educational Value of the Nursery School*. British Association for Early Childhood Education, London. (Still available from BAECE).

Jameson, Kenneth (1973). *Pre-school and Infant Art*. Studio Vista, London.

Kellogg, Rhoda (1955). *What Children Scribble and Why*. National Press, California.

Lindstrom, Miriam (1957). *Children's Art*. University of California Press.

Matterson Elizabeth (1989). *Play with a Purpose for the Under Sevens*, 3rd edn. Penguin, London.

Nutbrown, Cathy (1994). *Threads of Thinking: young children learning and the role of early education.* Paul Chapman, London.

Nutbrown, Cathy (1996) *Children's Rights and Early Education.* Paul Chapman, London.

Pugh, Gillian and De'Ath, Erica (1989). *Working Towards Partnership in the Early Years.* National Children's Bureau, London.

Helping Agencies and Their Addresses

ACTION FOR SICK CHILDREN
Argyle House, 29-31 Euston Road, London NW1 2SD (0171 833 2041; fax 0171 837 2110)

ADVISORY CENTRE FOR EDUCATION (ACE)
1b Aberdeen Studios, 22 Highbury Grove, London N5 2DQ (0171 354 8318; fax 0171 354 9069)

ADVISORY COUNCIL FOR THE EDUCATION OF ROMANY AND OTHER TRAVELLERS (ACERT)
Moot House, The Stow, Harlow, Essex CM20 3AG (01279 418666)

AFRICAN ASSOCIATION FOR MATERNAL AND CHILD CARE INTERNATIONAL (AAMCCI)
Family Connection Centre, Adunola Lodge, 13 Tatam Road, London NW10 8HT (0181 961 0268; fax 0171 624 6106)

AFRO CARIBBEAN EDUCATION RESOURCE PROJECT (ACER)
Acer Centre, Wyvil School, Wyvil Road, London SW8 2TJ (0171 627 2662; fax 0171 627 0278)

ALL WALES PLAY FORUM (AWPF)
c/o Dominique Wright (Secretary), Leisure & Amenities, Heath Park Offices, Cardiff CF4 4EP (01222 751235; fax 01222 822924)

ANTI BULLYING CAMPAIGN (ABC)
101 Borough High Street, London SE1 9QQ (0171 378 1446; fax 0171 378 8374)

ASSOCIATION FOR BRAIN DAMAGED CHILDREN AND YOUNG ADULTS
Clifton House, 3 St Pauls Road, Foleshill, Coventry CV6 5DE (01203 665450)

ASSOCIATION FOR FAIR PLAY FOR CHILDREN IN SCOTLAND
Unit 29, Six Harmony Row, Govan, Glasgow G51 3BA (tel & fax 0141 425 1140)

ASSOCIATION FOR POST NATAL ILLNES (APNI)
25 Jerdan Place, London SW6 1BE (0171 386 0868)

ASSOCIATION FOR SPINA BIFIDA AND HYDROCEPHALUS (ASBAH)	ASBAH House, 42 Park Road, Peterborough PE1 2UQ (01733 555988; fax 01733 555985)
ASSOCIATION OF BREASTFEEDING MOTHERS (ABM)	Sydenham Green Health Centre, 26 Holmshaw Close, London SE26 4TH (0181 778 4769)
ASSOCIATION OF PARENTS OF VACCINE DAMAGED CHILDREN	2 Church Street, Shipston on Stour, Warwickshire CV36 4AP (01608 661595)
BIRTH DEFECTS FOUNDATION (BDF)	Chelsea House, Westgate, London W5 1DR (0181 862 0198; fax 0181 991 5263)
BLACK CHILDCARE NETWORK	17 Brownhill Road, Catford, London SE6
BLISSLINK/NIPPERS	17–21 Emerald Street, London WCIN 3QL (0171 831 9393; fax 0171 404 0676)
BRITISH ASSOCIATION FOR EARLY CHILDHOOD EDUCATION (BAECE)	111 City View House, 463 Bethnal Green Road, London E2 9QY (tel & fax 0171 739 7594)
BRITISH ASSOCIATION FOR THE STUDY AND PREVENTION OF CHILD ABUSE AND NEGLECT (BASPCAN)	10 Priory Street, York YO1 1EZ (01904 613605; fax 01904 642239)
CAMPAIGN FOR STATE EDUCATION (CASE)	158 Durham Road, London SW20 0DG (tel & fax 0181 944 8206)
CHILD ACCIDENT PREVENTION TRUST (CAPT)	4th Floor, Clerks Court, 18–20 Farringdon Lane, London EC1R 3AU (0171 608 3828; fax 0171 608 3674)
CHILD BEREAVEMENT TRUST	1 Millside, Riversdale, Bourne End, Buckinghamshire SL8 5EB (tel & fax 01494 765001)
CHILD GROWTH FOUNDATION (CGG)	2 Mayfield Avenue, Chiswick, London W4 1PW (0181 995 0257/994 7625; fax 0181 995 9075)
CHILD POVERTY ACTION GROUP (CPAG)	4th Floor, 1–5 Bath Street, London EC1V 9PY (0171 253 3406; fax 0171 250 0622)

CHILDLINE	2nd Floor, Royal Mail Buildings, Studd Street, London N1 0QW (0171 239 1000)
CHILDLINE CYMRU	1a York Street, Swansea, West Glamorgan SA1 3LZ (01792 480111)
CHILDREN 1ST: ROYAL SCOTTISH SOCIETY FOR PREVENTION OF CRUELTY TO CHILDREN (RSSPCC)	Melville House, 41 Polwarth Terrace, Edinburgh EH11 1NU (0131 337 8539; fax 0131 346 4462)
CHILDREN'S RIGHTS OFFICE	235 Shaftesbury Avenue, London WC2H 8EL (0171 240 4449; fax 0171 240 4514)
COMMISSION FOR RACIAL EQUALITY (CRE)	Elliott House, 10–12 Allington Street, London SW1E 5EH (0171 828 7022; fax 0171 828 5680)
COUNCIL FOR AWARDS IN CHILDREN'S CARE AND EDUCATION (CACHE)	8 Chequer Street, St Albans, Hertfordshire AL1 3XZ (01727 847636/967333; fax 01727 867609)
COUNCIL FOR DISABLED CHILDREN (CDC)	National Children's Bureau, 8 Wakley Street, London EC1V 7QE (0171 843 6000; fax 0171 278 9512)
CRUSE BEREAVEMENT CARE	Cruse House, 126 Sheen Road, Richmond, Surrey TW9 1UR (0181 940 4818; bereavement line 0181 332 7227; fax 0181 940 7638)
CRY-SIS SUPPORT GROUP	BM CRY-SIS, London WC1N 3XX (0171 404 5011)
DISABLEMENT INFORMATION AND ADVICE LINES (DIAL UK)	Park Lodge, St Catherines Hospital, Tickhill Road, Doncaster DN4 8QN (01302 310123; fax 01302 310404)
DOWN'S SYNDROME ASSOCIATION (DSA)	155 Mitcham Road, London SW17 9PG (0181 682 4001; fax 0181 682 4012)
EARLY YEARS TRAINERS ANTI-RACIST NETWORK (EYTARN)	PO Box 1870, London N12 8JQ (0181 446 7056; fax 0181 446 7591)
EFFECTIVE PARENTING	117 Corringham Road, London NE11 7DL (0181 458 8404)
END PHYSICAL PUNISHMENT OF CHILDREN (EPOCH)	77 Holloway Road, London N7 8JZ (0171 700 0627; fax 0171 700 1105)
ENURESIS RESOURCE AND INFORMATION CENTRE (ERIC)	65 St Michael's Hill, Bristol BS2 8DZ (0117 926 4920; fax 0117 925 1640)

EQUAL OPPORTUNITIES COMMISSION (EOC)	Overseas House, Quay Street, Manchester M3 3HN (0161 833 9244; fax 0161 835 1657)
EQUALITY LEARNING CENTRE (ELC)	356 Holloway Road, London N7 6PA (0171 700 8127; fax 0171 700 0099)
EXPLORING PARENTHOOD	4 Ivory Parade, Treadgold Street, London W11 4BP (0171 221 4471; fax 0171 221 5501)
FAMILY NURTURING NETWORK	Bernwood Annexe, Bernwood First School, North Way, Headington, Oxford OX14 1 HJ (tel & fax 01865 744641)
FAMILY WELFARE ASSOCIATION (FWA)	501 Kingsland Road, Dalston, London E8 4AU (0171 254 6251; fax 0171 249 5443)
FOUNDATION FOR THE STUDY OF INFANT DEATHS (FSID)	14 Halkin Street, London SW1X 7DP (0171 235 0965; fax 0171 823 1986)
GINGERBREAD	16-17 Clerkenwell Close, London EC1R 0AA (admin. 0171 366 8183; advice line 0171 336 8184; fax 0171 336 8185)
GINGERBREAD NORTHERN IRELAND	169 University Street, Belfast, County Antrim BT7 1HR (01232 231417; fax 01232 240740)
GRANDPARENTS' FEDERATION	Room 3, Moot House, The Stow, Harlow, Essex CM20 3AG (01279 444964)
HIGH/SCOPE UK	Copperfield House, 190-192 Maple Road, London SE20 8HT (0181 676 0220; fax 0181 659 9938)
HOME-START UK	2 Salisbury Road, Leicester LE1 7QR (0116 233 9955; fax 0116 233 0232)
HYPERACTIVE CHILDREN'S SUPPORT GROUP (HACSG)	71 Whyke Lane, Chichester, West Sussex PO19 2LD (01903 725182)
KIDS' CLUBS NETWORK	Bellerive House, 3 Muirfield Crescent, London E14 9SZ (0171 512 2112; fax 0171 512 2010)
KIDSCAPE	152 Buckingham Palace Road, London SW10 9TR (0171 730 3300; fax 0171 730 7081)
LA LECHE LEAGUE (GREAT BRITAIN) (LLLGB)	BM 3424, London WC1N 3XX (0171 242 1278)

LETTERBOX LIBRARY (CHILDREN'S BOOKS LTD)	Unit 2D, Leroy House, 436 Essex Road, London N1 3QP (0171 226 1633; fax 0171 226 1768)
LONDON MONTESSORI CENTRE (LMC)	18 Balderton Street, London W1Y 1TG (0171 493 0165; fax 0171 629 7808)
LOW PAY UNIT	29 Amwell Street, London EC1R 1UN (0171 713 7616)
MEET-A-MUM ASSOCIATION (MAMA)	Cornerstone House, 14 Willis Road, Croydon CR0 1XX (0181 665 0357; fax 0181 665 1972)
MENCAP EARLY YEARS PROJECT (LONDON DIVISION)	115 Golden Lane, London EC1Y 0TJ (0171 608 2130; fax 0171 608 3254)
MUDIAD YSGOLION MEITHRIN (MYM)	145 Albany Road, Y Rhath, Caerdydd CF2 3NT (01222 485510; fax 01222 470196)
MULTIPLE BIRTHS FOUNDATION (MBF)	Queen Charlotte's and Chelsea Hospital, Goldhawk Road, London W6 0XG (0181 740 3519; fax 0181 740 3041)
NATIONAL ASSOCIATION FOR GIFTED CHILDREN (NAGC)	Park Campus, Northampton NN2 7AL (01604 792300; fax 01604 720626)
NATIONAL ASSOCIATION FOR SPECIAL EDUCATIONAL NEEDS (NASEN)	NASEN House, 4/5 Amber Business Village, Amber Close, Amington, Tamworth, Staffordshire B77 4RP (01827 311500; fax 01827 313005)
NATIONAL ASSOCIATION OF TOY AND LEISURE LIBRARIES (PLAY MATTERS)	68 Churchway, London NW1 1LT (0171 387 9592; fax 383 2714)
NATIONAL AUTISTIC SOCIETY (NAS)	276 Willesden Lane, London NW2 5RB (0181 451 1114; fax 0181 451 5865)
NATIONAL CHILDBIRTH TRUST (NCT)	Alexandra House, Oldham Terrace, London W3 6NH (0181 992 8637; fax 0181 992 5929)
NATIONAL CHILDMINDING ASSOCIATION (NCMA)	8 Masons Hill, Bromley, Kent BR2 9EY (0181 464 6164; fax 0181 290 6834)
NATIONAL CHILDMINDING ASSOCIATION IN WALES	Offices 4 & 5, The Lighthouse Business Park, Bastion Road, Prestatyn, Clwyd LL19 7ND (tel & fax 01745 852995)

NATIONAL CHILDREN'S BUREAU	8 Wakley Street, London EC1V 7QE (0171 843 6000; fax 0171 278 9512)
NATIONAL CHILDREN'S BUREAU, EARLY CHILDHOOD UNIT (ECU)	8 Wakley Street, London EC1V 7QE (0171 843 6000; fax 0171 278 9512)
NATIONAL COUNCIL FOR ONE PARENT FAMILIES (NCOPF)	255 Kentish Town Road, London NW5 2LX (0171 267 1361; fax 0171 482 4851)
NATIONAL COUNCIL FOR VOCATIONAL QUALIFICATIONS (NCVQ)	222 Euston Road, London NW1 2BZ (0171 387 9898; fax 0171 387 0978)
NATIONAL DEAF CHILDREN'S SOCIETY (NDCS)	15 Dufferin Street, London EC1Y 8PD (0171 250 0123; fax 0171 251 5020)
NATIONAL EARLY YEARS NETWORK	77 Holloway Road, London N7 8JZ (0171 607 9573; fax 0171 700 1105)
NATIONAL ECZEMA SOCIETY (NES)	163 Eversholt Street, London NW1 1BU (0171 388 4097; fax 0171 388 5882)
NATIONAL LIBRARY FOR THE HANDICAPPED CHILD	Reach Resource Centre, Wellington House, Wellington Road, Wokingham, Berkshire RG11 2AG (01734 891101; fax 01734 790989)
NATIONAL NEWPIN	Sutherland House, 35 Sutherland Square, London SE17 3EE (0171 703 6326; fax 0171 701 2660)
NATIONAL PLAYBUS ASSOCIATION (NPA)	93 Whitby Road, Brislington, Bristol BS4 3QF (0117 9775375; fax 0117 9721838)
NATIONAL PORTAGE ASSOCIATION (NPA)	127 Monks Dale, Yeovil, Somerset BA21 3JE (tel & fax 01935 71641)
NATIONAL SOCIETY FOR THE PREVENTION OF CRUELTY TO CHILDREN (NSPCC)	NSPCC National Centre, 42 Curtain Road, London EC2A 3NH (0171 825 2500; library enquiries 0171 825 2706; fax 0171 825 2525)
NATIONAL STEPFAMILY ASSOCIATION (STEPFAMILY)	Chapel House, 18 Hatton Place, London EC1N 8JH (0171 209 2460; fax 0171 209 2461)
NCH ACTION FOR CHILDREN	85 Highbury Park, London N5 1UD (0171 226 2033; fax 0171 226 2537)

NORTHERN IRELAND PRESCHOOL PLAYGROUPS ASSOCIATION (NIPPA)	Enterprise House, Boucher Crescent, Boucher Road, Belfast BT12 6HU (01232 662825; fax 01232 381270)
NORWOOD CHILD CARE (NCC)	Norwood House, Harmony Way, off Victoria Road, London NW4 2BZ (0181 203 3030; fax 0181 202 3030)
ONE PARENT FAMILIES SCOTLAND	13 Gayfield Square, Edinburgh EH1 3NX (0131 556 3899/4563; fax 0131 557 9650)
PARENT INFANT PROJECT (PIPPIN)	c/o Parent Network, 44–46 Caversham Road, London NW5 2DS (0171 485 8535)
PARENT NETWORK	44–46 Caversham Road, London NW5 2DS (0171 485 8535; fax 0171 267 4426)
PARENTING EDUCATION AND SUPPORT FORUM	8 Wakley Street, London EC1V 7QE (0171 843 6099)
PARENTLINE	Endway House, The Endway, Hadleigh, Benfleet, Essex SS7 2AN (01702 554782; fax 01702 554911)
PLAYGROUP NETWORK	PO Box 23, Whitley Bay, Tyne and Wear NE26 3DB (01912 521516)
PRE-SCHOOL PLAYGROUPS ASSOCIATION (PPA)	69 Kings Cross Road, London WC1X 9LL (0171 833 0991; fax 0171 837 4942)
RACE EQUALITY UNIT (REU)	5 Tavistock Place, London WC1H 9SN (0171 387 9681; fax 0171 387 7968)
REFUGEE COUNCIL	3 Bondway, London SW8 1SJ (0171 820 3000; fax 0171 582 9929)
ROYAL NATIONAL INSTITUTE FOR THE BLIND (RNIB)	224 Great Portland Street, London W1N 6AA (0171 388 1266; fax 0171 388 2034; education/family support fax 0171 383 4921)
ROYAL SOCIETY FOR MENTALLY HANDICAPPED CHILDREN AND ADULTS (MENCAP)	123 Golden Lane, London EC1Y 0RT (0171 454 0454; fax 0171 608 3254)
ROYAL SOCIETY FOR THE PREVENTION OF ACCIDENTS (RoSPA)	Cannon House, The Priory Queensway, Birmingham B4 6BS (0121 200 2461; fax 0121 200 1254)
RURAL DEVELOPMENT COMMISSION	19 Dacre Street, London SW1H 0DH (0171 340 2900)

SAVE THE CHILDREN (SCF)	17 Grove Lane, London SE5 8RD (0171 703 5400; fax 0171 703 2278)
SCOPE	12 Park Crescent, London W1N 4EQ (0171 636 5020; fax 0171 436 2601)
SCOTTISH CHILD LAW CENTRE	170 Hope Street, Glasgow G2 2TU (0141 333 9305; fax 0141 353 3861)
SCOTTISH CHILDMINDING ASSOCIATION (SCMA)	Room 7, Stirling Business Centre, Wellgreen, Stirling FK8 2DZ (01786 445377; fax 01786 449062)
SCOTTISH PRE-SCHOOL PLAY ASSOCIATION (SPPA)	SPPA Centre, 14 Elliot Place, Glasgow G3 8EP (0141 221 4148; fax 0141 221 6043)
SENSE, THE NATIONAL DEAFBLIND AND RUBELLA ASSOCIATION	11–13 Clifton Terrace, Finsbury Park, London N4 3SR (0171 272 7774; fax 0171 272 6012; minicom 0171 272 9648)
SHELTER	88 Old Street, London EC1V 9HU (0171 253 0202)
SIA: THE NATIONAL DEVELOPMENT AGENCY FOR THE BLACK VOLUNTARY SECTOR	High Holborn House, 49–51 Bedford Row, London WC1V 6DJ (0171 430 0811; fax 0171 831 9767)
SICKLE CELL SOCIETY	54 Station Road, Harlesden, London NW10 4BO (0181 961 7795)
SOLDIERS' SAILORS' AND AIRMEN'S FAMILIES ASSOCIATION (SSAFA)	SSAFA Central Office, 19 Queen Elizabeth Street, London SE1 2LP (0171 403 8783; fax 0171 403 8815)
STILLBIRTH AND NEONATAL DEATH SOCIETY (SANDS)	28 Portland Place, London W1N 4DE (0171 436 7940; fax 0171 436 3715)
TWINS AND MULTIPLE BIRTHS ASSOCIATION (TAMBA)	PO Box 30, Little Sutton, South Wirral L66 1TH (tel & fax 0151 348 0020)
WALES PRE-SCHOOL PLAYGROUPS ASSOCIATION (WALES PPA)	2a Chester Street, Wrexham, Clwyd LL13 8BD (01978 358195; fax 01978 312335)
WORKING GROUP AGAINST RACISM IN CHILDREN'S RESOURCES (WGARCR)	Lady Margaret Hall, 460 Wandsworth Road, London SW8 3LX (0171 627 4594; fax 0171 622 9208)

WORLD ORGANISATION FOR EARLY CHILDHOOD EDUCATION (OMEP)
c/o A. Lewis, 144 Eltham Road, London SE9 5LW (0181 850 3981)

CENTRAL GOVERNMENT DEPARTMENTS

DEPARTMENT FOR EDUCATION AND EMPLOYMENT
Sanctuary Buildings, Great Smith Street, London SW1P 3BT (0171 925 5000; Library 0171 925 5189; TASC [Teaching as a career] 0171 925 6616)
The former Department of Employment offices remain at Caxton House, Tothill Street, London SW1H 9NF (0171 273 3000)

DEPARTMENT OF HEALTH
Richmond House, 79 Whitehall, London SW1A 2NS (0171 210 3000) also Wellington House, 133–155 Waterloo Road, London SE1 8UG (0171 972 2000)

Index

Abuse 9, 64–7
Accidents
  accident book 62
  contributing factors 54–5
  involving blood 33–4
  prevention in the home 55–7
  see also Safety
Acquired immunity 30
Active immunity 30–1
Acute asthma attack 37
Additives 77–8
Addresses, useful 201–9
Adult
  role in play 166–9
  to child ratio, outings 60
Aesthetic and creative areas of learning, under
      fives 191
AIDS 44, 45–7
  see also HIV infection
Airborne spread of infection 29
Alcohol, ante-natal care 87
Allergies 81
  and additives 77–8
  and weaning 104
Alpha-fetoprotein 91
Amniocentesis 91
Anaemia
  sickle cell disease 49
  thalassaemia 50
Ante-natal
  care 86–9
  screening 89–92
Anti-bias curriculum and good practice 17–20
Anti-discriminatory practice 10
Anti-racist curriculum 19–20
Anti-stereotyping, resources 10, 15, 181
Antibodies 30

Antitoxins 30
Apgar score 93–4
Artificial immunity
  active 31
  passive 31
Asian community, rickets and osteomalacia 48
Assignments
  child development 163
  child health 53
  diet and nutrition 83
  play and education 198
  safety 62, 63, 68
  working with babies 117
  working with children 20
Asthma 37–8

Babies
  care of 105–17
  safety 50–1, 58, 113, 116
  working with 84–117
Bacteria 28
Bacterial infections
  dysentery 27
  scarlet fever 27
  skin 47
  whooping cough 26
Bandura, child development theory 125
Bathing 108–10, 130
Bathroom/toilet, accident prevention in 56–7
Battered child syndrome 64
Bedroom, accident prevention in 57
Behavioural
  effects of poverty 7
  indicators
    physical abuse 67
    sexual abuse 67
  patterns and reinforcement 125

Birth 92–3
Birthmarks 97–8
Block play 175–6
Blood, accidents involving 33–4
Blood screening, ante-natal 89–90
Bonding with carers 84–5
Book corner 181
Books 180–2
Bottle feeding 102–4
    preparing feed 102–4
    reasons for 100
Breast feeding 100–1
    nipple position 101
    reasons for 99–100
Bruner, child development theory 125, 132

Calcium 75
Calories 71
Carbohydrates 72
Carers see Child care workers; Parents
Carriers, infectious diseases 29
Changing nappies 105–8
Chickenpox 25, 29
Child
    abuse see Abuse
    care costs 4
    development see Development
    health see Health
    protection, role of carer 67–8
    safety see Safety
Child care workers
    attitude to parents 116–17, 196–7
    response, disclosures of abuse 68
    responsibilities in event of accident 63
    role in child protection 67–8
Children Act 1989, children in need 16
    HIV positive children 47
    see also Special needs
Children, working with 1–20
Child's role in society 1
Chorion biopsy 91
Clay, playing with 185–6
Cleaning, preventing spread of infection 34
Clearing away activities 190
Clothing for outings 58
Coeliac disease 38
Cognitive development 111–12

Collection, children from nursery or playgroup 64
Common
    childhood illnesses 36–50
    infectious diseases of childhood 24–7
Common cold 24, 29
Confidentiality
    'at risk' status 67
    HIV/AIDS 46, 47
    observations and assessments 194
Congenital dislocation of hip, examination of
        newborn 95
Conjunctivitis 29, 38
Conservation test, child development 160
Constructive/manipulative play 174–5
Convulsions 38
Cookery activities 154, 186–8
Coryza 24, 29
Costs
    average weekly per child 7
    child-care 4
Cot death, reducing risk 58, 110–11
Cradle cap 42, 47
Creative
    development, learning outcomes, pre-school
        children 196
    play 176–80
Cultural aspects, child development 120–2
Curriculum
    anti-bias and good practice 17–20
    anti-racist 19–20
    early years 190–4
    hidden 11–17
Cystic fibrosis 38–9, 44

Dance 182–3
Date-stamps, pre-packaged foods 81–2
Daytime naps 52
Dehydration 72
Dental care, ante-natal 88
Department of Health
    guidance, cot deaths 1991 58
    hygiene procedures 1992 32–4
Dermatitis 40–2
    seborrhoeic 42, 47
Development 119–63
    babies, stimulation and 111–16
    stages in painting 178–80

theorists 122-5
through play 170-3
Development, stages of 113-15, 125-63
  1-3 months 125-8
  3-6 months 128-31
  6-9 months 131-3
  9-12 months 133-6
  15-18 months 136-40
  18-24 months 140-3
  2½-3 years 143-8
  3-4 years 148-53
  4-5 years 153-6
  5-6 years 156-9
  6-7 years 159-61
  7-8 years 161-2
Developmental delay, signs
  6-8 months 133
  at 12 months 136
  at 18 months 140
  at 6 years 161
Diabetes mellitus 39-40
Diarrhoea 40
Diet and nutrition 70-83
  ante-natal 87-8
  feeding new baby 99-105
  mother's for breast feeding 101
  nutritional information 71-8
Diplococcus 28
Direct spread of infection 29
Disability 16-17
Diseases
  common childhood illnesses 36-50
  infectious 24-7
Disposable nappies 105
Disposal of waste 34
Domestic violence 9-10
Down's syndrome, prenatal diagnosis 91
Dreams and nightmares 52
Dressing up 154
Droplet, spread of infection 29
Drugs, ante-natal care 88-9
Dysentery 27, 29

E numbers 77-8
Early years curriculum 190-4
Eczema 40-1
Education and play 165-98

Emergency situations 62-3
Emotional abuse 65
Emotional development
  1-3 months 127
  3-6 months 130-1
  6-9 months 132-3
  9-12 months 135-6
  15-18 months 139
  18-24 months 142
  2½-3 years 147-8
  3-4 years 151-2
  4-5 years 156
  5-6 years 158
  6-7 years 160
  7-8 years 162
  through play 171
Energy value of food 71
Environmental factors, accidents 55
Equal opportunities 17-18
  promoting 10-17
Equipment
  setting out 189-90
  storing 190
Erikson, child development theory 123-5
Ethnic minorities
  parents in play and education 197
  unemployment 8
Exercise 52
  ante-natal care 88
Extended family 2-3
Eyes, reflexes of newborn 96

Face, examination of newborn 95
Failure to Thrive (FTT) 42-7, 50
  indicators of potential 43
Families
  different types of 2-5
  factors mitigating against 5-10
  violence within 9-10
    see also Abuse
Fantasy play 173
Fats 73
Febrile convulsions 38
Feely books 180
Fetal abnormality, screening tests for 90-2
Fibre 73
Figures, drawing 179-80

Fire drills 62
First aid 62–3
First trimester 86, 87
Food
    additives *see* Additives
    allergies 77–8, 81, 104
    hygiene 81–2
    introducing new foods 79–80, 104–5
    preparing, play and education 186–8
Food Handling Certificate 81
Formula, bottle feeding 102
Freud, child development theory 123
Froebel, Friedrich 165
Fruit, preparation of 82
Fungal infections, ringworm 48
Fungi 28

Garden, accident prevention in 57
Gasteroenteritis 27, 29, 40, 104
Gender stereotyping 12–13, 153
General measures, preventing spread of
        infection 33
Genitals, examination of newborn 95
German measles 26, 89
Glue ear 43
Grasp reflex, newborn 96, 126
Grave concern 65

Haemophilia 43–4
Hands and feet, examination of newborn 95
Head and neck, examination of newborn 95
Head Start programme 192
Headlice 44–5
Health 23–53
    see also Diet and nutrition
Health and development, factors essential 23
Hearing, newborn 97
Heart, examination of newborn 95
Helping agencies, addresses 201–9
Hepatitis 45
Heuristic play 115–16
Hidden curriculum 11–17
Highscope 112, 192
HIV infection 44, 45–7
    prevention of spread, Department of Health
        guidelines 32–4

Home life and social class 5–6
Homelessness 8–9
Houses, drawing 179–80
Human factors, accidents 54–5
Human and social areas of learning, under fives 191
Hygiene
    basic routine 35–6
    Department of Health guidelines 32–3
    food 81–2
Hyperactivity 77–8
Hyperglycaemia 39–40
Hypoglycaemia 39

Illness
    common childhood 36–50
    dealing with sick child 36
    multi-cultural aspects 24
    signs of 36
    see also Infections
Imaginative play 168, 173–4, 193
Immunity, types of 30–1
Immunization 30, 31–2
    schedule 32
Impetigo 29, 47
Indirect spread of infection 29
Infections 24
    body's defences 30
    common infectious diseases of childhood 24–7
    spread of 28–9
Infectious diseases, prevention of spread,
        procedures 35–6
    Department of Health 32–4
Influenza 29
Ingestion, spread of infection 29
Inhalation, spread of infection 28–9
Injury sites, accidental and non–accidental 66
Inoculation, spread of infection 29
Integration, children with special needs 16, 17
Intellectual development
    1–3 months 126–7
    3–6 months 129–30
    6–9 months 132
    9–12 months 134
    15–18 months 138–9
    18–24 months 141
    2½–3 years 145–6
    3–4 years 149, 149–51

4-5 years 154-5
5-6 years 157-8
6-7 years 159-60
7-8 years 162
Piaget's stages of 122-3
through play 170-1
Interest tables 188
Intra-uterine infection 29
HIV 46
Iodine 75-6
Iron 76

'Junk' foods 71
Junk table, items for 177

Kidscape 64
Kitchen
accident prevention in 55-6
hygiene 82
Knowledge and understanding of the world,
learning outcomes, pre-school children 196

La Leche League 101
Labelling 11, 12-13
see also Stereotyping
Labour, stages of 92-3
Landers, Cassie, definition of culture 120
Language
newborn 97
race, colour and ethnicity 15
social class and home life 5-6
Language development
1-3 months 126, 127
3-6 months 130
9-12 months 134-5
15-18 months 139
18-24 months 141-2
2½-3 years 146-7
3-4 years 151
4-5 years 115-16
5-6 years 158
6-7 years 160
through play 171-2
Language and literacy
areas of learning, under fives 191

learning outcomes, pre-school children 196
Learning outcomes 169, 194-6
Listening skills, children's 183
Listeria 88
Lone parent families 4
Lounge, accident prevention in 56
Low income 4
impact on diet and nutrition 70-1
see also Poverty
Lymphatic system 30

Manipulative/constructive play 174-5
Materials
for imaginative play 174
for junk table 177
Mathematics
areas of learning, under fives 191
learning outcomes, pre-school children 196
Mealtimes 78-81
weaning 105
Measles 25, 29
Measurements, examination of newborn 95
Meningitis 28
Menus for nurseries 80
Microwave ovens 82
Milia 98
Minerals 75-7
Mixed Failure to Thrive 42
Moles 98
Mongolian blue spot 98
Monosaturated fats 73
Montessori, Maria 193
Moral areas of learning, under fives 192
Moro reflex, newborn 96, 97, 126
Mother, ante-natal screening 89-90
Movement 182-3
Multi-cultural aspects, children's illnesses 24
Multiple births, prenatal diagnosis 92
Mumps 25-6, 29
Music 182-3
Musical instruments 183

Nappy
changing 105-8
rash 47, 108
Naps, daytime 52

National Occupational Standards for Working with Under Sevens and their Families 1-2
Natural immunity
    active 30-1
    passive 31
Neglect 65
Neonatal urticaria 98
New foods, introduction of 79-80, 104-5
Newborn 93-4
    abilities of 97
    examination of 95-9
    reflexes 96, 97, 125, 126
Nightmares and dreams 52
Nipple position, breast feeding 101
Non-accidental injury *see* Physical abuse
Non-Organic Failure to Thrive 42
Norms within family 2, 5, 9
NSPCC, definitions of abuse 64-5
Nuclear family 3-4
Nutrition *see* Diet and nutrition

Observations
    activities 169
    and assessment, early years curriculum 194
    development 120
Oral reflex, newborn 96
Organic Failure to Thrive 42
Organization
    of activities 168-9
    outings 59-61, 189
Osteomalacia 48
Outings
    clothes for 58
    organization and planning 59-61, 189
    safety on 58-62
Over-stimulation 127

Painting 178
    stages of development in 178-80
Parents
    care of babies 116-17
    education, involvement in 196-8
Passive immunity 31
Personal hygiene, food handling 82
Personal and social development, learning
        outcomes, pre-school children 196

Pertussis 26
Phosphorus 76
Physical abuse 65
    indicators of 66-7
Physical areas of learning, under fives 192
Physical development
    1-3 months 125-6
    3-6 months 128-9
    6-9 months 131-2
    9-12 months 133-4
    15-18 months 136-8
    18-24 months 140-1
    2½-3 years 143-4
    3-4 years 148-9
    4-5 years 153-4
    5-6 years 156-7
    6-7 years 159
    7-8 years 161
    fine motor movements 135
    learning outcomes, pre-school children 196
    small muscle control 138
    through play 170
Physical effects, poverty on children 7
Piaget, child development theory 122-3, 139
Pigmented naevi 98
Planning play activities 188-9
    see also Organization
Plastic pants 106
Play
    activities, setting out and clearing away 188-90
    development through 170-3
    and education 165-98
    role of adult in 166-9
    value of different types 173-88
Pneumonia 28
Poetry 182
Poliomyelitis 29
Polyunsaturated fats 73
Port Wine Stain 98
Portage system 193-4
Potassium 76
Poverty 6-8
    diet and nutrition 70-1
    long term consequences 7
    see also Low income
Pregnancy, signs and stages 86
Premature babies 96-7
Protein 72

Psychosexual development, Freud's stages of 123
'Pygmalion in the Classroom', Rosenthal and
    Jacobson 12-13

Questions
    children's 168
    open ended 167-8

Race, culture and ethnicity 15
    see also Ethnic minorities; Skin colour, signs and
        symptoms of illness
Rashes
    chickenpox 25
    eczema, characteristics of 41
    measles 25
    nappy 47, 108
    newborn 98
    rubella 26
    scarlet fever 27
Reconstituted families 3, 4-5
Records
    accident book 62
    child's progress 194
    contact numbers 62
Reflexes, newborn 96, 97, 125, 126
Refrigerators 81
Reinforcement and behaviour 125
Resources
    anti-bias curriculum 17
    anti-stereotyping 10, 15, 181
Respiratory tract infections 29
Rest and sleep 50-2
    babies' sleep patterns 111
    daytime naps 52
    sleeping arrangements 50-1
Rhymes 182
Rickets 48
Right and left handedness 138-9
Ringworm 48
Road safety 59
Role play 173-4
Rooting reflex, newborn 96
Rosenthal and Jacobson (1968) 'Pygmalion in the
    Classroom' 12-13
Routines
    bathing a baby 108-10

bottle feeds 102-4
nappy changing 106-8
pre-mealtime 78
Rubella 26
    ante-natal care 89
Rumbold Committee (DES, 1990), early years
    curriculum 191

Safety 54-68
    abuse 64-7
    babies 50-1, 58, 113, 116
    dealing with strangers 63-4
    in the home 55-8
    outside the home 58-62
    setting out equipment 189
    see also Accidents
Salmonella 82, 88
Sand play 184-5
Saturated fats 73
Scapegoating 12-13
Scarlet fever 27, 28
Scenarios
    anti-bias curriculum 19
    child development 149, 153, 156, 159
    childhood illnesses 40, 44, 47
    dealing with aggressive behaviour 16
    diet and nutrition 72, 75, 81
    homelessness 10
    infectious diseases 28
    play and education 169, 183, 186, 197
    safety 57
    step-parenting and behaviour problems 12
    working with babies 85, 91, 99
Schema, Athey (1990) 167
Scientific and technological areas of learning, under
    fives 192
Screening
    ante-natal 89-90
    for fetal abnormality 90-2
Scribbling 179
Seborrhoeic dermatitis 42, 47
Second trimester 86
Sexual abuse 65
    indicators of 67
Sick child, dealing with 36
Sickle cell disease 48-50
Single-parent families 4

Sitting room, accident prevention in 56
Skin colour and signs and symptoms of illness 24
Sleep and rest 50-2
   babies' sleep patterns 111
   daytime naps 52
   sleeping arrangements 50-1
Small-for-dates babies 97
Smell, newborn 97
Smoking, ante-natal care 87
Snacks 80
Social class and home life 5-6
Social development
   1-3 months 128
   3-6 months 131
   6-9 months 133
   9-12 months 136
   15-18 months 139-40
   18-24 months 142-3
   2½-3 years 148
   3-4 years 152-3
   4-5 years 156
   5-6 years 158-9
   6-7 years 160-1
   7-8 years 162
   Erikson's theory 123-5
   through play 172-3
Social learning theories 123-5
Society, child's role in 1
Sodium 76
Solids, introduction of 104-5
Space, concept of 150-1
Special needs 16
   disability 16-17
   learning outcomes 169
   mealtimes 81
   Portage system 193-4
Spina bifida, pre-natal diagnosis 91
Spiritual areas of learning, under fives 192
Spots and rashes *see* Rashes
Stages of development *see* Development, stages of
Staphylococcus 28
Startle reflex 96, 97, 126
Steiner, Rudolph 192-3
Step-parents 3, 4-5
Stereotyping 10, 11, 12, 13-14, 153
Sterilization
   bottle feeding 102, 103-4
   terry towelling nappies 106

Stimulating babies 111-16
Stork's beak marks 98
Storytelling 180-2
   traditional stories 181-2
Storytime 181
Strangers, dealing with 63-4
Strawberry marks 98
Streptococcus 28
Sudden infant death syndrome *see* Cot death,
     reducing risk
Symbolic play 173

Table manners 79
Teacher's expectations of children 13
   'Pygmalion in the classroom' experiment 12-13
Temperature
   babies room 110
   refrigerators 81
Temporary accommodation, children living in
     8-9
Terry towelling nappies 105-6, 106-8
   folding 107
Thalassaemia 50
Third trimester 86
Thrush 108
Time, concept of 149-50
Tinea 48
Toilet training 143
Toilet/bathroom, accident prevention in 56-7
Touch, newborn 97
Traditional stories 181-2
Transport for outings 61
Treasure basket, heuristic play 115-16

Ultrasound, ante-natal screening 90
Umbilical cord, examination of newborn 95
Unemployment 6-7, 8
Urine, ante-natal screening 90

Value system of the home 2, 5, 9
Vegetables, preparation 82
Vegetarian diets 72, 80
   ante-natal care 88
Violence, family 9-10
   see also Abuse

Viral infections
  chickenpox 25
  common cold 24
  measles 25
  mumps 25–6
  rubella 26
Viruses 28
Vision, newborn 97
Vitamins 73–5
  A 73
  B complex 73–4
  C 74
  D 48, 74–5
  E 75
  K 75
Von Willebrand's disease 43

Waldorf education system 192–3

Walking reflex, newborn 96
Waste, disposal of 34
Water
  dietary 72
  play 183–4
Weaning 104–5
Whooping cough 26
Women, role in extended family 3
Working
  with babies 84–117
  with children 1–20
World Health Organization (WHO), child health
    and development 23

X-rays, ante-natal care 89

Zinc 76–7